"Mind-body approaches are generally neglected in clinical medicine, and almost no one thinks of using them in the treatment of diabetes. Dr. Surwit is a welcome exception. In this book he explains how to take advantage of the mind-body connection to control blood sugar in ways that are less expensive, less toxic, and as effective as conventional approaches."
—ANDREW WEIL, M.D.

"Dr. Richard Surwit, the world's leading expert in diabetes and the mind-body connection, has written the premier guidebook to living a healed, whole and healthy life with diabetes."
—JOAN BORYSENKO, Ph.D., author of *Minding the Body,*
Mending the Mind and *Inner Peace for Busy Women*

"Dr. Surwit shows that diabetes has a mind of its own—in other words, stress can raise the blood glucose higher than all the dietary indiscretions and indulgence that most humans allow themselves. With Dr. Surwit's easy-to-follow program for managing stress and depression, people with diabetes can conquer their demons and take charge of their health. A must-read for physicians and their patients."
—LOIS JOVANOVIC, M.D., Director and Chief Scientific Officer,
Sansum Medical Research Institute

"I highly recommend that all health care professionals and people with diabetes learn Dr. Surwit's methods of stress management and make them part of their diabetic care."
—CLIFTON BOGARDUS, M.D., internationally
recognized diabetes researcher

"A world-renowned expert and pioneer in understanding the interaction of behavior and diabetes, Dr. Surwit presents great mind-body strategies for managing the disease and keeping blood glucose under better control. *The Mind-Body Diabetes Revolution* is also a pleasure to read, and individuals who use it as part of their diabetes self-care program increase their chances of living better and longer lives."
—STEVEN E. LOCKE, M.D., President, American Psychosomatic Society;
Associate Professor of Psychiatry, Harvard Medical School

"This is an outstanding book! Drawing upon his decades of experience working with diabetic patients, Dr. Surwit has given us not only a practical and useful step-by-step approach for achieving control of diabetes, but also an inspiring road map to mental well-being."
—PATRICK LUSTMAN, Ph.D., Professor of Psychiatry
at Washington University School of Medicine, St. Louis

"The specific steps aren't difficult to add to your daily routine and may make just the difference you've been hoping for."
—AMAZON.COM

The Proven Way to Control Your Blood Sugar by Managing Stress, Depression, Anger and Other Emotions

The
MIND-BODY
Diabetes
Revolution

Richard S. Surwit, Ph.D.

with Alisa Bauman

Foreword by Jay S. Skyler, M.D.

MARLOWE & COMPANY
NEW YORK

THE MIND-BODY DIABETES REVOLUTION:
The Proven Way to Control Your Blood Sugar by Managing Stress, Depression, Anger and Other Emotions
Copyright © 2004, 2005 by Richard S. Surwit, Ph.D., and Alisa Bauman
Foreword copyright © 2004 by Jay S. Skyler, M.D.

AVALON
publishing group incorporated

Published by
Marlowe & Company
An Imprint of Avalon Publishing Group Incorporated
245 West 17th Street • 11th Floor
New York, NY 10011-5300

Originally published in hardcover by Free Press, a Division of Simon & Schuster, Inc. This edition published by arrangement.

The Library of Congress has cataloged the hardcover edition as follows:

Surwit, Richard S.
The mind-body diabetes revolution: a proven new program for better blood sugar control/Richard S. Surwit, with Alisa Bauman.
p. cm.
Includes bibliographical references and index. 1. Diabetes—Treatment—Popular works. 2. Diabetes—Psychological aspects—Popular works. 3. Behavior therapy. I. Bauman, Alisa. II. Title.
RC660.S87 2004   616.4'6206—dc22   2003063146

ISBN 0-7432-4991-7

This edition ISBN 1-56924-363-8

9 8 7 6 5 4 3 2 1

Designed by Karolina Harris
Printed in the United States of America

Dedicated to my grandparents, who suffered with diabetes for many years and died prematurely because of this disease

Contents

Foreword

For more than twenty years, I've closely followed Richard Surwit's research into the connection between stress and diabetes. I first learned of his research during the early 1980s, when I heard of work that he was performing with his colleague Mark Feinglos. Their first study suggested a possible link between stress and blood glucose control. I was intrigued. They told me about dramatic transformations in some of their patients with diabetes. The stories whetted my appetite; I wanted to know more. I learned that in that study, Dr. Surwit had taught a simple relaxation technique to six patients with diabetes. Another six patients with diabetes had served as a control group and had not learned the relaxation technique. After just one week, those who learned the relaxation technique had improved glucose control compared to those who did not learn to relax.

That small study led to larger studies, which led to other studies in mice and additional studies on human beings. Now, more than twenty years later, Richard Surwit is considered one of the foremost experts on the connection between stress and diabetes. He has published scores of studies on the topic.

Dr. Surwit's work has revealed that stress is indeed a crucial determining factor in diabetes control. That's not all. More recent research done by his team, as well as by other researchers across the country, shows that additional psychological factors also play a role in blood glucose control. These additional factors include depression and hostility.

Psychological factors such as stress, depression, and hostility are considered as detrimental to the progression of diabetes as a poor diet. Dr. Surwit has studied and fine-tuned psychological techniques that help people with diabetes overcome stress and other mental problems that aggravate their condition. The results have been dramatic. In some cases, patients have had improvement in diabetic complications. In others, they were able to get their blood glucose under control when all else had failed.

Although the importance of psychological factors in diabetes control is well recognized by many experts in the field, including myself, it is still difficult for patients with diabetes to receive appropriate psychological treatment. Most small diabetes clinics do not offer it, and many insurance companies will not pay for it. *The Mind-Body Diabetes Revolution* takes this program at Duke University out of the lab and into the homes of millions of people with diabetes. With this book, this important program is now accessible to all who need it.

In *The Mind-Body Diabetes Revolution,* Dr. Surwit explores how thoughts and beliefs influence our emotions and moods and can result in anger, depression, and anxiety. The book will help you find out whether the state of your mind is negatively affecting your diabetes. You'll take a series of tests to find out whether you are suffering from undue stress, depression, or hostility. You will discover that relaxation and cognitive behavior exercises can lead to a healthier mind, which can result in such physical changes as weight loss and improved blood glucose control.

Then you will learn simple, proven techniques to help reduce stress, lift depression, and ease hostility. You'll learn the techniques one step at a time over six weeks. After six weeks, you'll have made them a habit and will be able to call on your arsenal of psychological techniques when you need them.

This program is no substitute for standard treatment. You still must follow a healthful diet. You still must exercise and take prescribed medication. This program is, however, a way for you to get your blood glucose under control, especially if nothing else has worked. It will teach you how to use your mind to help heal your body. It's a very simple yet powerful addition to your diabetes treatment plan. I recommend that you embark on the program today.

JAY S. SKYLER, M.D.

Past President, American Diabetes Association;
Professor of Medicine, Pediatrics, and Psychology and
Director of the Division of
Endocrinology/Diabetes/Metabolism,
University of Miami

Preface to the Paperback Edition

Since the initial publication of *The Mind-Body Diabetes Revolution* in March of 2004, several important new studies have been published that add support to the main ideas presented in this book. In May of 2004, the world-renowned medical journal, *The Lancet,* published a large meta-analysis (a study of studies) of twenty-five studies examining the effects of a variety of psychological techniques on blood sugar levels.[1] This study concluded that these techniques—the same ones outlined in this book—do indeed lower blood sugar in people with diabetes. On average, patients participating in programs designed to reduce psychological distress showed a 0.75 percent reduction in hemoglobin A1c, which is a reliable marker for average blood sugar. That's a significant reduction, one equal to that of many diabetes medications.

When I first wrote *The Mind-Body Diabetes Revolution,* I noted that depression and diabetes seemed interconnected. The current research at that time, however, did not effectively show which people with diabetes—type 1 versus type 2—could most benefit from psychological techniques to lift depression. Now we have that research. In a large study involving over 1,000 people with both type 1 and type 2 diabetes,[2] my lab found that depression seems to have a particularly negative effect on blood sugar in patients with type 1 diabetes who take three or more insulin injections a day! This reinforces the notion that controlling symptoms of depression may be helpful for this specific subset of patients.

Not only is there now more evidence for the importance of managing psychological distress, but we now have conclusive evidence that simply eliminating caffeine can produce a significant improvement in glucose tolerance in patients with diabetes. In a study headed up by Dr. James Lane at Duke and published in *Diabetes Care*[3] in August of 2004, eliminating caffeine reduced the blood sugar increase following a meal by 21 percent! This change is as large as changes reported for several new oral diabetes medicines!

That research, along with the research already outlined in this book, proves that the psychological techniques in *The Mind-Body Diabetes Revolution* can help people with diabetes control blood sugar. That said, the real beauty to the *The Mind-Body Diabetes Revolution*'s methods is this: they are safe, free of side-effects, and once you learn the techniques outlined in this book, they are yours to use and enjoy for life!

I have received much positive feedback from readers of the hardcover edition of *The Mind-Body Diabetes Revolution* over the past year. Many people report that this book has made a very positive change in their lives in general, as well as specifically in their blood sugar control. I sincerely hope you find this book as useful.

RICHARD S. SURWIT, PH.D.

Durham, North Carolina

NOTES

1. Ismail, K. et al. Systematic review and meta-analysis of randomized controlled trials of psychological interventions to improve glycaemic control in patients with type 2 diabetes. *Lancet,* 2004, 363; 1589–1597.
2. Surwit, RS. et al. Treatment regimen determines the relationship between depression and glycemic control. *Diabetes Research and Clinical Practice,* 2005, 69, 78–80.
3. Lane, JD. et al. Caffeine impairs glucose metabolism in type 2 diabetes. *Diabetes Care,* 2004, 27, 2047–2048.

Introduction

I'm very pleased that you've decided to embark on a journey to better health with the *Mind-Body Diabetes Revolution*.

As a medical researcher, I often cringe when I see the word *revolution* attached to any new therapy, diet, or technique. Yet research into the mind-body connection in diabetes has grown so strong and so convincing over the past twenty years that we can no longer ignore it. Indeed, we now know that the mind and the body are intricately linked. We also know that you can use the powers of your mind to influence your body in profound ways, including normalizing blood sugar levels.

Since you've bought this book, you probably have diabetes or you're concerned that you may develop it. And you've probably been told to do three things: watch your diet and lose weight, exercise, and possibly take medication.

The treatment of diabetes has changed little over the past forty years. Although many new medications have been developed, patients still must watch their diets closely, exercise, and take insulin or oral medications throughout the day. And in spite of adhering to a strict treatment regimen, many continue to struggle to control their blood sugar.

Recognizing the mind-body connection and how it affects blood sugar provides a fourth vital element in diabetes treatment. What goes on inside your head and inside your brain and mind can affect your body in profound ways. Taking a few simple steps to change your mental outlook can dramatically improve your health and your diabetes, often bringing the most stubborn cases of high blood sugar under control.

Although the mind-body connection to diabetes is well understood among medical researchers, this is the first book to present it to people outside the laboratory, to those who need it most: people who have diabetes or may be at risk for developing it. It's not that there's a conspiracy among physicians or health educators to keep this information from you. Most physicians are trained to prescribe medications or counsel you about your diet and exercise habits. Many aren't trained in the mind-body techniques suggested throughout the pages in this book, techniques that we at Duke University have studied, developed, and proven to work.

I decided to write this book at the urging of many physicians and health educators who want the program that we developed and tested at Duke in writing so that they can use it to teach others. The major impetus came not long ago when one of my studies about the connections between stress and blood sugar appeared in *Diabetes Care* and generated quite a bit of attention.

In the study, we had asked 108 people with type 2 diabetes to undergo five diabetes education sessions with or without stress management training. During the stress management sessions, patients learned progressive muscle relaxation as well as other techniques to help them cope with stress. After one year, those who followed the program experienced a 0.5 percent improvement in HbA_{1C} (a type of blood protein that indicates whether a person's average blood sugar levels are normal). Although that sounds like a very small reduction in blood sugar, this small degree of change is enough to reduce risk significantly for diabetes-related complications such as eye and kidney disease. Furthermore, nearly a third of the people in the study experienced much larger improvements, of 1 percent or more. Most compelling was that the technique worked for everyone, including those who initially didn't report that stress was a major factor in their lives.

The study built on research that I had been doing for twenty years, so I was somewhat surprised by the media response. Almost as soon as the study appeared, I was flooded with phone calls from reporters. Popular magazines, radio programs, and TV news broadcasts brought the news from our labs at Duke into the homes of millions of people across the country. Then more calls began pouring in—these from people with diabetes and people who treat those with diabetes. They wanted to know if they could purchase materials to help them learn the program we had tested.

We scrambled to help. We sent out the audiotape and booklet that we had used in the study to hundreds of callers. As we struggled to keep up with demand, the idea for *The Mind-Body Diabetes Revolution* was born.

The Mind-Body Diabetes Revolution is based on the research that I and many others have done, linking psychological factors such as stress and depression to blood sugar control. Everything suggested in this book has been shown in scientific studies to be effective. That said, *The Mind-Body Diabetes Revolution* is no substitute for traditional diabetes treatment, such as medication, exercise, and a proper diet. Rather, it is an important complement to those treatments. If you've struggled to get your blood sugar under control with other methods, I believe that *The Mind-Body Diabetes Revolution* may provide the extra bit of help you need.

The Mind-Body Diabetes Revolution can help you improve your outlook on life and lift your mood. It can help you to stick to important lifestyle habits such as a proper diet. It provides the important final ingredient to your blood sugar control arsenal, helping to lower your blood sugar levels once and for all. Even if your blood sugar is already under control, the program will help provide some extra insurance, particularly on those days when you may not attend to your dietary or physical needs as well as you should.

In Part I, you'll learn about the mind-body connection in diabetes. You'll follow my research that links stress, depression, and hostility to blood sugar control and find out why the mind-body connection is so important to your health.

In Part II, you'll learn what to do with this new understanding. You'll first take a few crucial tests to determine your psychological state. Based on your answers, you'll then choose to learn one of two mind-body techniques—or you can decide to learn both. I'll guide you in how to put them together into a six-week program. For example, if your tests reveal that you feel very stressed but not depressed or angry, you will focus on just one mind-body technique: progressive muscle relaxation. If your tests find that depression or anger is your major problem, you will focus on a different mind-body technique: cognitive behavior therapy. If your tests show that you feel angry *and* stressed, you will combine the techniques. I present each technique in six simple steps, and you can tackle each slowly and gradually over six weeks.

In Part III, you'll find an optional mind-body program, based on the skills you learned in Part II, that will help you control your appetite and lose weight. You'll also learn about additional mind-body techniques that have been shown to improve blood sugar control. And you'll learn about important medications and common substances that may help or hinder your success on *The Mind-Body Diabetes Revolution* programs. You'll also find contact information for mind-body resources and various organizations where you can expand your learning beyond the pages of this book.

The techniques explained in this book have been tested by men and women from many different ethnic backgrounds and walks of life. I've found that they are applicable to everyone, regardless of age, race, religion, sex, or education.

I'm confident that you too will find the tools you need in these pages. And by using this program, you will do more than improve your blood sugar control; you will also improve your outlook on life. After six weeks with the program, you can expect to feel comfortable with your new techniques, and your blood sugar control will begin to improve. If you stick with the program, you should see changes in your health and your general sense of well-being.

Congratulations on your decision to explore your mind-body connection, the fourth important element in blood sugar control. Let's get started.

Part I

Your Mind's Healing Power

1
Understanding Diabetes

Manage the Emotions That Can Aggravate
Your Condition

Two of my grandparents had diabetes. My father's father had
diabetes from the time he was a young man and died at the age
of fifty-nine, when I was only two years old. My mother's mother
came down with it in her fifties. I still remember my grandmother, who died when I was ten, giving herself insulin shots.

Both my grandfather and grandmother died of heart disease,
the major cause of death among patients with diabetes. Because
both of these grandparents were immigrants and raised their
families during the Great Depression, they attributed their diabetes to the terrible stress of their lives, so I too always assumed
that diabetes was somehow related to stress.

Now, many years later, I earn my living as a stress researcher.
I have spent the best part of the past thirty years trying to
understand how stress affects the development, progression,
and resolution of illness. During my graduate studies at McGill
University and postdoctoral studies at Harvard Medical School,
I studied how stress affects high blood pressure, migraine
headache, and Raynaud's disease (poor blood flow in the fingers and toes).

In the late 1970s, shortly after I moved to Duke, I ran into a
young endocrinologist, Mark Feinglos, who had also studied at
McGill. He wanted to know if I had any psychological techniques that might be useful for treating diabetes. I had com-

pletely forgotten about diabetes, the disease that had killed my grandparents and the disease for which I likely carried at least some of the genes. Although I had assumed that stress was as important in diabetes as my grandparents thought, I did not really know it to be true scientifically. I decided to find out.

Working with Dr. Feinglos, I set out on a research program that has spanned almost a quarter-century. My research group and others at universities around the world have conducted numerous studies on thousands of patients and animals to understand better how stress and other psychological factors influence this disease. The results of this research have proven that my grandparents were right: *stress, depression, and a person's general psychological state greatly influence blood sugar in every individual with diabetes. These mental states may even determine whether genetically susceptible people develop diabetes in the first place.*

Although research on the importance of psychological factors has been published in the top scientific journals, it has not found its way into most diabetes treatment programs. To this day, most people with diabetes are still treated with the same three program components that have been used for the past fifty years: diet, exercise, and medication. Patients are provided with some training in nutrition, told to exercise regularly, and given oral medicine or insulin, or both. Few treatment programs address the important psychological factors involved in blood sugar control.

The Mind-Body Diabetes Revolution gives you the fourth important component of diabetes treatment in a detailed step-by-step program. You'll learn how to use the power of your mind to control your body better. The psychological techniques in this program have been proven at Duke University Medical School and elsewhere to improve blood sugar control, and the different components of this program have been tested in clinics around the country in studies involving hundreds of patients. We have shown over and over again that once you know why your blood sugar remains high, you will be able to address the emotions that may aggravate your condition.

Before we get into the program, let's first take a closer look at your *metabolism,* the rate at which your body burns up or uses blood sugar (glucose).

YOUR METABOLISM 101

Diabetes is quickly becoming the nation's biggest health crisis. It affects nearly 20 million people. Since you're reading this book, you've probably already been diagnosed with diabetes or are concerned that you may develop it. A family history of diabetes is one of the strongest indicators of whether you will get the disease. To see if you may be at risk for developing diabetes, take a moment to contemplate the following facts:

- If one of your parents developed type 2 diabetes before age fifty, your risk of developing diabetes is 1 in 7. (See box, Diabetes 101, for a definition of "type 2" and "type 1.")
- If one of your parents developed type 2 after age fifty, your risk of developing diabetes is 1 in 13.
- If both of your parents had type 2, your risk of developing diabetes is 1 in 2.
- If your father had type 1, your risk of developing diabetes is 1 in 17.
- If your mother had type 1 and you were born before she turned age twenty-five, your risk of developing type 1 diabetes is 1 in 25.
- If your mother had type 1 and you were born after she turned age twenty-five, your risk of developing type 1 diabetes is 1 in 100.

To get your blood sugar under control, you first must understand the inner workings of your cells, hormones, and organs. You also must understand that what's wrong inside your body is not your fault. Blaming yourself and feeling guilty can actually worsen the condition by making you feel depressed and anxious. To prove to you that you didn't cause your condition, let's take a journey deep inside your body.

Often one of the first symptoms of diabetes mellitus is frequent urination, produced by high blood sugar. Ancient physicians noticed that in patients with this condition, the urine often tasted sweet (hence, *diabetes,* meaning frequent urination, and *mellitus,* meaning honey). Diabetes develops when body cells cannot process glucose, a simple sugar that serves as the primary fuel for all cells in the body. Your body converts most of the food you eat into glucose, fats, and proteins during the process of digestion before burning it as fuel. Let's say you just ate a meal. You chew your food and break it down in your mouth, mixing it with saliva. You swallow. Blood vessels in your mouth, stomach, and intestines absorb the sugar from your food into your bloodstream.

Your pancreas, an organ below your stomach, senses this rise in blood sugar. This important organ responds by secreting substances that aid digestion and several hormones, including the hormone insulin. Produced in clusters of beta cells in your pancreas called the islets of Langerhans, insulin helps control your metabolism. In a healthy person, the beta cells in the pancreas send out just enough insulin to allow the blood sugar to be processed by the body as needed.

Insulin acts like a key to unlock the doors of muscle and other body cells and allow glucose in. If you eat more food than your body requires at the time, insulin allows this excess energy to be stored by the liver, muscles, and fat cells. In people with diabetes, however, something goes wrong. In people with type 1 diabetes, the beta cells in the pancreas are destroyed by the body's own immune system and can no longer produce any insulin.

In type 2 diabetes, the problem is somewhat more complex. The pancreas produces insulin—sometimes more than normal. But the insulin doesn't work properly. It's as if the cells in your body have all changed their locks, and insulin can't get them to open their doors and let in the sugar. This is called *insulin resistance,* and it's often how diabetes starts. The result is the same: the sugar remains in the blood in high concentrations, setting you up for a number of health problems.

When you have insulin resistance, your pancreas senses that

your blood sugar is high and responds by producing even more insulin. Scientists believe that either this constant strain on the pancreas or the chronically elevated blood sugar itself can wear out your pancreas, which becomes unable to release enough insulin to regulate blood sugar. Ultimately, many patients with type 2 diabetes develop an inability to produce normal amounts of insulin.

Whatever has gone wrong inside your body, the blood sugar doesn't get to where it needs to go. It remains high in the blood for longer than normal. Though your kidneys eventually flush the sugar out into your urine, high blood sugar brings on a host of problems.

DIABETES 101

Diabetes refers to a series of disorders that affect blood sugar levels:

PREDIABETES. Also called glucose intolerance, prediabetes means that your blood sugar is higher than normal but not high enough to place you in the diabetic category. About 16 million people have prediabetes (17 million have full-blown diabetes).

METABOLIC SYNDROME. Also called syndrome X, this refers to several conditions that often occur together. They include obesity, insulin resistance, diabetes or prediabetes, hypertension, and high blood cholesterol.

TYPE 1 DIABETES. Type 1 diabetes is an autoimmune disease where your immune system attacks the beta cells (insulin-producing cells) in your pancreas and wipes them out over a period of time. It develops during childhood and makes insulin shots a necessity.

TYPE 2 DIABETES. Type 2 tends to develop in adults and used to be called adult-onset diabetes. Today, however, younger and younger people, including teenagers, are developing the disease. This type of diabetes is really a spectrum of different diseases. For some people, the pancreas overproduces insulin, and cells fail to respond to it. (See *insulin resistance* below.) In others, cells respond normally to insulin, but the pancreas doesn't secrete enough of it, because the pancreas doesn't completely sense the correct blood sugar level.

INSULIN RESISTANCE. This refers to your body's inability to use the insulin it produces. Lack of exercise, obesity, and a high-fat diet make insulin resistance more likely.

HYPERINSULINEMIA. This may start with an overproduction of insulin, which may encourage cells to stop recognizing the hormone, which leads to producing even more insulin. High insulin levels increase your tendency to store fat, so they contribute to obesity as well.

THE COST OF HIGH BLOOD SUGAR

High blood sugar triggers health problems in the kidneys, eyes, heart, and nerves. Several studies have shown that blood sugar may be even more important than cholesterol levels or blood pressure in predicting heart disease and premature death. In fact, blood sugar is a major contributor to other ailments, such as high blood cholesterol and stroke. Many people who die of heart disease may have gotten those clogged blood vessels from mildly elevated blood sugar.

High blood sugar damages both large and small blood vessels, although exactly how it does so is not well understood. In the large blood vessels, high blood sugar spurs on the process of atherosclerosis, in which vessels harden and narrow as they become clogged with fatty plaques. In the small vessels, such as those found in the eyes and kidneys, high blood sugar produces leakage and bleeding. For these reasons, diabetes is the leading cause of blindness, kidney disease, and limb amputations. Specifically, here's how diabetes affects certain conditions:

• NERVE DISEASE. High blood sugar seems to damage the nerves, which can cause numbness, pain, and tingling anywhere in the body. When high blood sugar damages nerves around the organs, it alters the message relay system between the brain and organs. For example, nerves in the digestive tract may fail to tell the intestines to contract, which can cause constipation and incontinence. Damage to the nerves controlling the heart can leave diabetic patients susceptible to dangerous heart rhythm changes that lead to sudden death. Diabetes-induced nerve damage is also a leading cause of impotence in men.

• HEART DISEASE. People with diabetes are two times more likely to suffer a heart attack as those without it. This is particularly risky in women with type 2, who have a three to four times higher risk of heart disease than women without diabetes. Diabetes increases levels of fats circulating in the blood, which get stuck along the linings of arteries, creating plaque that can eventually clog the arteries. Stiffer, narrowed blood vessels make the heart work harder to pump blood, which raises blood pressure. Higher pressure causes more damage to the arteries, creating a vicious cycle.

• STROKE. People with diabetes are two times more likely to suffer a stroke as those without it. As blood sugar levels rise, blood becomes thicker, increasing the chances of a stroke. Just as blood vessels surrounding the heart can narrow and become damaged by high blood sugar, so can the smaller blood vessels in the brain. High blood pressure, which is also associated with high blood sugar, weakens arteries in the brain, causing them to bleed.

• EYE DISEASE. Diabetes is the leading cause of blindness, and half of those with diabetes develop eye disease. People with diabetes are twenty times more likely to go blind than those without it. When the blood vessels in the eyes get damaged from high blood sugar, they weaken and leak, damaging the retina and clouding vision. Eventually, this can even destroy eyesight.

• KIDNEY DISEASE. Diabetes is the leading cause of kidney failure: people with diabetes are forty times more likely to suffer kidney failure than those without it. With diabetes, the kidneys must work overtime to filter excess sugar out of the blood. Eventually, the blood sugar destroys the cells in the kidney that filter the blood. In addition, many people with diabetes also have high blood pressure, which further damages the kidneys.

• DIABETES. High blood sugar damages the pancreas, so it is possible that patients whose blood sugar that runs in the high-normal range may be damaging their pancreas and pushing themselves further toward diabetes. For those who have diabetes, high blood sugar also eventually destroys the beta cells that secrete insulin.

Blood sugar is not the only culprit in diabetes. High insulin levels, or hyperinsulinemia, common in early type 2 diabetes, may be as bad as high sugar levels. Excess insulin may also damage the heart, blood vessels, and nerves, and it can increase blood pressure.

AS SERIOUS AS CANCER

Many people don't take diabetes seriously. Your doctor may have diagnosed you with diabetes after you complained of seemingly benign symptoms. Perhaps you felt more fatigued than usual or had frequent headaches. Until it starts to hurt your health, the condition seems more like a nuisance than an actual threat.

On death certificates, diabetes is rarely listed as the cause of death. Instead, people who die with diabetes are said to have died of kidney failure, heart attack, stroke, and other organ diseases. Nonetheless, those diseases were probably caused by diabetes.

The good news is that research done in the last ten years has shown that keeping tight control of your blood sugar can help reduce and possibly even eliminate these health consequences. So whereas many people live in dread of cancer, diabetes may actually be worse than cancer for some people. *Diabetes significantly decreases life expectancy.* Many people with cancer may actually be able to live longer than people with diabetes. The difference between cancer and diabetes is that, with appropriate medication and lifestyle change, you can do more to manage your disease than someone with cancer can.

If you've discounted the serious ramifications of diabetes, you're not alone. Until recently, even the medical and scientific community paid little attention to type 2 diabetes. For most of the twentieth century, researchers focused on ways to cure type

1 diabetes, the type that develops during childhood. The discovery of insulin in the 1920s allowed children with type 1 to live into adulthood. Even so, because regular insulin shots don't completely mimic the natural rises and falls of insulin, blood sugar is still hard to control, and people with type 1 often die prematurely of diabetic complications.

Until recently, type 2 diabetes, which tends to develop in adulthood, garnered little attention. Since the 1990s, however, the number of people affected by the disease has skyrocketed. (I'll explain why in a minute.) Today, type 1, which affects about 500,000 people in the United States, seems like a minor public health problem compared with type 2, which affects close to 20 million Americans and is growing rapidly in the United States and around the world. In fact, type 2 diabetes is starting to affect children, something unheard of just a decade ago.

Diabetes isn't just an American problem. It is a world health crisis. Experts have predicted that the Chinese will have 200 million people with type 2 diabetes by 2020, with India close behind.

WHEN NORMAL ISN'T NORMAL

Those grave numbers reflect only people with full-blown diabetes. Countless numbers of other people have a condition we now call *prediabetes,* and still others are genetically prone to diabetes but have not yet developed the disease. And still other people who test normal on typical blood sugar exams at a physician's office and who technically don't have "diabetes" have day-to-day blood sugar levels that are high enough to increase their risk of serious health complications.

Your blood sugar level is vitally important to your well-being. Many people probably have higher average blood sugar levels than they should, and most people don't know it. Unlike blood pressure and cholesterol, doctors rarely check blood sugar levels unless the patient reports diabetes-like symptoms. That's why the American Diabetes Association estimates that as many as 5 million people have undiagnosed diabetes.

As more and more research emerges on the health risks of

poor blood sugar control, we're learning that what we once thought of as a normal reading may still raise the risk for disease. Blood sugar levels include a large gray area between what's considered healthy and what's considered diabetic. The lower your average blood sugar levels are, the lower is your risk for disease. The higher your levels, the higher your risk is.

In years to come, we may learn more precisely what constitutes a truly "normal" or "healthy" blood sugar level. For now, this is what we consider normal, prediabetic, and "diabetic":

NORMAL: Fasting blood sugar less than 110 mg/dl; blood sugar two hours after a meal less than 140. (Fasting blood sugar is a reading taken at least eight hours after eating. Blood sugar rises after you eat. Some people have high fasting blood sugar levels and normal post-meal blood sugar levels—and vice versa—so it's important to know both readings.)

PREDIABETIC: Fasting blood sugar between 110 and 125; blood sugar two hours after a meal between 140 and 200

DIABETES: Fasting blood sugar over 125; blood sugar two hours after a meal over 200

THRIFTY GENES: YOUR GENETIC DESTINY

Diabetes is a frustrating disease. You may be doing everything right to control your blood sugar: you watch what you eat, exercise, and may even be taking medication. Yet your blood sugar may still remain out of control.

Both type 1 and type 2 diabetes are complex disorders. Certain genetics make some people more prone to diabetes than others. But even for people with such genetics, something in the environment seems to trigger the onset of diabetes. For instance, if one identical twin has type 1 diabetes, there's a 50 percent chance that the other twin will develop it too, but we don't yet know why one develops the disease while the other does not.

The genetics of type 2 diabetes are probably a bit more complicated than type 1, but we have a somewhat better understanding of how genetic predisposition interacts with environment in type 2. We think that the most common varieties of type 2 diabetes and its cousins, obesity and insulin resistance, come from what's called a *thrifty genotype*. This hypothesis was first developed in 1962 by a scientist named James V. Neel to explain why some animals and people seem to be predisposed to develop obesity and diabetes. Here is the idea, briefly stated:

As little as 100 years ago, thrifty genes helped people survive. Nearly every society around the globe led an existence characterized by periodic feasts and famines. The poor survived on potatoes, rice, and bread. Meat and cheese were considered luxuries. Calories were scarce. As a result, people tended to be much smaller and leaner than they are today. People who had the "thrifty" genotype tended to survive such harsh living conditions and pass on their genetics.

In the past, women whose bodies were able to store more fat during lean times tended to get pregnant and lactate, passing on their thrifty genes to their offspring. Women whose bodies tended to burn calories at a high rate and not store fat usually couldn't get pregnant during lean times, so they didn't pass on their genetics. This is why obesity genes are so common. It is also why most fertility symbols in primitive societies were figurines of obese women. Our ancestors knew that obese women could produce and raise children.

Your fat cells are actually endocrine cells that secrete a hormone called leptin. The fatter you are, the higher your leptin level is. Leptin has many different roles in controlling body weight, including regulation of appetite and metabolic rate. It also tells the brain whether there is enough stored energy to allow a woman to become fertile. Women with very low body fat, such as some athletes, and women with severe eating disorders cannot become pregnant. Leptin is nature's way of preventing a woman from having a baby she can't feed.

Over the thousands of years of human civilization, this feast-or-famine existence has resulted in more and more people today possessing not just one but many genes related to diabetes. In fact, societies that lived through feasts and famines most recently have the highest rates of diabetes today. African

Americans, Native Americans, Asians, Polynesians, Aborigines, and Latin Americans now have the highest rates of diabetes. They have a strong genetic predisposition developed after years of starvation and subsistence on few calories and very little fat. As these societies switch to an Americanized lifestyle, with its excess fat and calories and a decrease in physical activity, they are also suffering greater rates of diabetes.

The Pima Indians provide a perfect example. Until the early 1900s, the Pimas lived off the land, farming and fishing. Living in the Southwest desert, they battled frequent droughts, sometimes feasting, sometimes starving. Those who survived such harsh conditions tended to have the ability to store fat when food was available. As little as 100 years ago, Pimas were a lean race of people in whom diabetes was rare.

When settlers destroyed the agrarian lifestyle that the Pima Indians had used to survive, during the early 1900s, they began to starve. The federal government began supplying lard and other high-fat foods to the Pimas. Today on the reservations, food is as plentiful as anywhere else in the country, and like many other Native Americans, the Pimas have exchanged their active lifestyle for a relatively sedentary one. Today, nearly 100 percent of Pimas are obese, and over 50 percent have type 2 diabetes, one of the highest rates in the world. Their genetics haven't changed, but their lifestyles have.

A group of researchers led by Dr. Eric Ravussin, then at the National Institutes of Health, found a group of Pima Indians living across the border in Mexico. They were the genetic cousins of the Arizona Pimas, but they had retained their traditional agrarian ways: they exercised more and ate far fewer calories. Few of these people were obese, and diabetes was practically nonexistent. This proves the important effects lifestyle has on obesity and diabetes.

Here's another example. At Duke, we've done quite a bit of research on mice (which share 80 percent of human genes) to help us understand the genetics of diabetes and obesity. We have found that like humans, different strains of mice carry different numbers of thrifty genes. When fed a low-fat diet, most strains of mice are lean and have normal blood sugar levels. Certain strains of mice, however, are genetically prone to balloon and develop diabetes as soon as the fat content of their diet is raised to the relative level that most Americans consume (40 percent calories from fat or more).

According to the thrifty gene theory, a number of different genes work together to slow the metabolism, promote fat storage, spike blood sugar and insulin, and make cells resistant to insulin. Over time, many different thrifty genes have evolved, each contributing to the thrifty genotype in a slightly different way. It's unlikely that one or even several genes will be discovered and deemed completely responsible for diabetes and obesity. Many genes are involved.

If you have one or more of the thrifty genes, your body may respond by:

- Turning down your metabolism and slowing calorie burning
- Making your cells resistant to insulin, so that sugar and fat can't get inside your cells to be burned for energy
- Overproducing insulin, which creates a one-way door for fat cells that allows them to store fat but makes it hard to get rid of it

Research from my own laboratory has shown that chronically high insulin levels, common in early diabetes, shut down the body's ability to burn fat, which lowers overall calorie-burning capability. High insulin levels block the body's ability to release fat stores. Consequently, high insulin levels have been linked to obesity and the development of type 2 diabetes.

The relationship between the body's tendency to store fat and its susceptibility to develop diabetes is well known, but we do not completely understand how fat storage leads to diabetes. The most likely explanation is that the more fat one stores, the more fat can compete with glucose as a fuel in most cells, causing a surplus of glucose to remain in the blood. As a result, the body suffers chronically from high blood sugar.

Exactly how severe your diabetes becomes depends largely

on how many thrifty genes you have, how much you exercise, and how and what you eat. Some people can control their blood sugar simply by watching what they eat or by losing weight. Others may need to add exercise to the mix. And still others may have so many thrifty genes that nothing—not even oral medication—will get blood sugar completely under control. These people often require additional insulin even if their pancreas is still working.

No matter how badly you've been walloped by genetics, however, there's still hope. Even if you never completely control your blood sugar, every little bit you do helps to slow the progression of complications.

THE FATTENING OF AMERICA

Calories are plentiful in this country. The cheapest food in America tends to be highest in calories and fat. In the 1800s, the poor lived on potatoes and rice. In the 2000s, the lower socioeconomic groups eat junk food and fast food. Family-style and fast food restaurants supersize their meals, making it possible for an individual customer to consume thousands of calories in just one meal consisting of a soda, fries, and a burger. That's two to three times the calories you need. I'm no exception even though I certainly know better. Not long ago, I was traveling with my family. We got to the airport around dinnertime and had an hour to kill so we walked around the airport looking for something to eat. There were no nutritious choices, and we eventually settled on fried chicken. When we got to Philadelphia, my daughter said she was still hungry. A McDonald's was within walking distance of our hotel, so we went there, and she ordered fries, which my wife and I nibbled on too. The restaurant was packed with teenagers who were drinking sodas and eating fries, loading up on hundreds of excess calories and fat. But my family and I do this only occasionally. For many Americans, this is a daily diet, setting them on the road to gaining weight and developing diabetes.

Type 2 diabetes will never go away all by itself. Our bodies will never genetically alter themselves to adjust to our new lifestyles.

Because type 2 diabetes does not usually develop until after people reach reproductive age, diabetes genes will not be weeded out of the population by evolution. People with type 2 rarely die before childbearing age. People with one or more thrifty genes continue to pass on their genetics.

The genes that promote the disease will continue to cause diabetes in humans for generations to come.

WHAT TO DO ABOUT YOUR BLOOD SUGAR

The life-changing program in this book will help you use your mind to manage your blood sugar better. That said, this program is no substitute for the three old standbys in diabetes treatment: diet and weight loss, exercise, and medication. Let's take a closer look at each.

Diet and Weight Loss

High-protein, high-fat diets are probably dangerous for people with blood sugar problems. Many people with diabetes may have some kidney problems, and high-protein diets, which stress the kidneys, can be very harmful. As it turns out, people with blood sugar problems generally do well on high-carbohydrate diets—as long as the fat content is very low. Our research at Duke has clearly shown that high-carbohydrate, low-fat diets will quickly lower blood sugar and promote weight loss. Patients on such diets have found them to be very effective for controlling diabetes.

Our research at Duke has also shown that blood sugar problems arise only when simple carbohydrates and fat are mixed together. Fat taxes the pancreas and induces hyperinsulinemia and insulin resistance, allowing the simple carbohydrates to raise blood sugar.

I suggest you follow a low-fat diet. It will help you manage your blood sugar and is better for your overall long-term health. Some people with diabetes do just fine on the American Heart Association's 30 percent fat diet, but the best results for most people with diabetes are found in diets that restrict fat even further, such as the programs of Dean Ornish, Pritikin, and the Rice

Diet. These diets usually obtain less than 10 percent of their calories from fat.

If you have diabetes, you may have heard that you should eat foods that are low on the glycemic index. The *glycemic index* is a measure of how fast your body absorbs the food you eat and raises blood sugar levels. The body absorbs simple carbohydrates such as sugar, potatoes, and rice very rapidly, which is why these foods are high on the glycemic index. The body absorbs high-fiber carbohydrate foods more slowly and protein and fats even more slowly. These foods are lower on the index.

For people with diabetes, lower-glycemic-index foods usually lead to lower blood sugar levels after a meal, which is why some people have suggested that overconsumption of high-glycemic-index foods leads to high insulin levels and diabetes. Research does not support this theory. Many studies have shown that if the fat content in the diet is low enough (usually less than 10 percent), very-high-glycemic-index foods have no adverse effects on blood sugar, insulin, or weight. In one study that we conducted at Duke, we fed overweight women either a low-fat diet consisting of 50 percent calories from sucrose (table sugar), which has a very high glycemic index, or no sugar at all. After six weeks, both groups lost the same amount of weight and had the same blood sugar and cholesterol levels. Furthermore, people with diabetes who went on the Rice Diet, which consists of numerous high-glycemic-index foods but very little fat, regularly lose weight and improve their blood sugar levels. So as long as you keep fat to a minimum, you probably do not have to worry about the glycemic index.

If you are overweight, however, you will want to lose a few pounds. This is usually easy to do on a very low-fat diet. Losing as little as 5 to 10 percent of your total weight may dramatically improve your blood sugar control by making your cells more sensitive to insulin. This will help preserve the beta cells in your pancreas. To do so, you must eat fewer calories than your body burns for energy. Once you lose the weight, you must eat roughly the same number of calories that your body burns. It's really a simple formula.

The weight-loss industry has a terrible track record, with most people quickly regaining whatever weight they lose. Most people succeed in losing weight, but they don't keep it off. Part of this failure stems from unrealistic goals. Rather than aiming to reach a "healthy" weight, most people strive for a "cosmetic" weight loss, which is often impossible to achieve. They therefore become discouraged and give up. If you weigh 200 pounds, you may need to lose only 10 to 20 pounds to improve your blood sugar. But most people who weigh 200 pounds try to lose much more—50, 60, 70, or more pounds. This type of goal is hard to maintain.

To succeed at weight loss, you must aim for a healthy weight. To get there, you must follow a program that you can maintain. The only way to keep the weight off is by keeping up the habits that you used to lose the weight in the first place. You'll find a mind-body program to help you lose weight in Chapter 10.

Exercise

Regular exercise helps lower blood sugar for numerous reasons. First, it helps you to burn more calories than you eat. Second, exercise helps you deal with stress and boost your mood, which, as you'll learn in coming chapters, is key in keeping blood sugar under control. Third, regular exercise improves your health and prevents some of the complications that occur with diabetes, such as heart disease.

Both aerobic exercise and strength training are important for people with diabetes. Aerobic exercise is the most effective way to burn calories and is also important in preventing heart disease. Strength training will increase your muscle mass, which increases your resting metabolism and makes your cells more sensitive to insulin. This in turn will lower your overall blood sugar and insulin levels, which allow your body to burn fat more easily. Lower insulin levels will also decrease your appetite.

If you have diabetes, it is critical that you consult your doctor before you begin any exercise program or diet program. You need to know that your body will tolerate what you are about to start, and you should have your doctor monitor your progress to make sure that it is having the desired effect on your condition.

Medication

Diet and exercise may not be enough to bring blood sugar under control. That's where medication comes in. Over the past ten years, numerous new medications have become available that can make a major difference in diabetes control. You need to take medication if diet and exercise don't work for you. Further, if you have diabetes, you should make sure that you are receiving the correct medication that you require. If in doubt, consult a diabetes specialist. You can find one by a referral from your regular doctor or through the American Diabetes Association (1-800 DIABETES or www.diabetes.org). You'll also find some helpful information about diabetes medications in Chapter 11.

WHY THIS PROGRAM WILL HELP

My first diabetic patient was Janice, whom I met many years ago when she was in the hospital because of severe complications from diabetes. She was on medication and had been doing everything right, but her diabetes was not responding. Within a week, I taught her the program that you will learn in this book. By the end of the week, her blood sugar was under much better control. Since then, I've taught hundreds of other patients the same technique with similar results.

The program works by tapping into your mind-body connection. As early as the seventeenth century, the famous physician Thomas Willis attributed the onset of diabetes to a problem with the nerves. Over the past hundred years, we have learned that the hypothalamus controls most metabolic functions. Hormones released from this area of the brain control appetite, metabolic rate, fat storage, and blood sugar. The key hormones involved in controlling blood sugar are also the key players in the body's response to stress. Thus, by controlling your response to stress, you can help regulate your metabolic control.

Though you cannot simply will your blood sugar to normal,

your metabolism is not beyond your control. You can learn certain techniques that will help put you in the right frame of mind for optimal blood sugar levels. By learning to take yourself from an anxious to a relaxed state, from a depressed mood to a happy one, from an angry state to a calm one, you can significantly influence blood sugar control.

The Mind-Body Diabetes Revolution will give you a little wiggle room. Adding psychological strategies to your current regimen will help you mentally relax a little and allow you to enjoy life more without suffering blood sugar surges as a result. It can even help you finally get blood sugar under control when all else has failed. Remember that you will still have to stay on your strict diet and take any medication that is prescribed for you.

Turn to Chapter 2 to discover the power of your mind and metabolism connection.

2

The Mind-Metabolism Connection

Why Psychological Techniques Can Help You
Control Your Blood Sugar

DURING the 1960s, researchers made a number of exciting discoveries about the inner workings of the human body. Until that time, physiologists had split bodily functions into two groups: voluntary processes that you could control, such as moving your arms and legs, and involuntary processes that you could not, such as your heartbeat, sweat rate, or immune system. Such involuntary processes, which normally run automatically, were thought to be beyond voluntary control. As we began to learn a few decades ago, however, that assumption wasn't completely accurate.

In a classic experiment of that time, Harvard researcher David Shapiro trained people to increase or decrease their sweat rate, their blood pressure, or heart rate based on feedback they received from a machine that measured these responses. When someone successfully lowered his or her sweat rate or blood pressure, the machine responded with a light, a tone, or a pleasing picture. Shapiro's work changed how scientists and health professionals viewed involuntary bodily functions. With the aid of what came to be known as *biofeedback,* patients could learn to control their blood pressure, sweating, and other so-called *autonomic* bodily processes.

I was just finishing my doctorate in clinical psychology at McGill University in Montreal when I became aware of Shapiro's work, which I found extremely exciting. I felt as if an entirely new universe has just been discovered. Biofeedback and this new field of mind-body research promised to revolutionize medicine and psychology, and I wanted to be among the first to explore it. So I wrote to Dr. Shapiro and applied to be a post-doctoral fellow at his laboratory in Harvard Medical School.

At Harvard, I joined the ranks of a small but growing number of researchers who studied animals and humans, trying to find out what other so-called involuntary responses—skin tempera-ture, heart rate, gastrointestinal response, brain chemistry, pain, metabolism, and even bleeding—could be controlled voluntar-ily. For instance, researchers tried to condition rats to raise the skin temperature of one ear and not the other. We also began looking into how we could harness the power of the mind to lower blood pressure, warm the hands and feet in people with circulation problems, and reduce headaches.

These and other studies have demonstrated that the brain can in part influence almost all body functions—even the immune system. During the 1970s, Robert Ader, a scientist at Rochester School of Medicine and Dentistry, made an accidental discovery that led to this understanding. Ader was trying to con-dition rats to avoid sugar-flavored water by adding to it a drug commonly used in chemotherapy that made them nauseous whenever they drank it. The method worked well. The rats needed only one experience with the sugar water and nausea to avoid the water for good. In addition to making the rats nause-ated, the drug also suppressed their immunity, an unforeseen side effect. In later experiments, Ader noticed that the rats suf-fered a drop in immunity whenever they encountered the sugar water, even when they weren't given the drug.

Ader had accidentally conditioned the rats' immune systems to respond to the sugar water. Further studies showed that the immune system was intimately connected to the nervous system.

THE POWERS OF THE MIND

Around this time, other scientists were discovering that emo-tional stress could worsen heart disease and blood pressure and even hinder conception. We researchers studied numerous relaxation techniques—some new, some old (techniques that you'll learn in Chapters 7 and 12)—that could activate the mind to help relieve headaches, prevent heart disease, and ease digestive problems. At Harvard, several of us began looking into how these relaxation techniques might be used to help those with Raynaud's disease, which causes poor blood flow to the fingers and toes and makes them hypersensitive to cold temperatures. We had heard stories of Buddhist monks in Tibet who could alter their skin temperature during meditation and withstand extremely cold temperatures without covering their bodies with clothing. It seemed too good to be true. The body naturally is supposed to reduce blood flow (and heat) to the extremities when cold and bring it to the center of the body to protect the vital organs.

To find out more, one of my colleagues, Herbert Benson, M.D., traveled to Tibet to study these monks. He had been part of the original group at Harvard working with Shapiro and realized that a simple meditation technique could produce the same effects as biofeedback, without the need for complex machinery. Later, in his classic book, *The Relaxation Response* (1975), Benson showed how people could use meditation to help themselves with many different medical conditions.

In Tibet, Benson studied the Buddhist monks to see how well they could control bodily functions. He tested three different monks. To see if they could truly control their skin temperature, Benson placed thermometers on each monk's body to measure skin and internal temperature as he meditated. As each monk entered a state of deep meditation, his skin temperature increased.

We in the United States were discovering the same ability in our own subjects. By using the biofeedback machines pioneered by David Shapiro, we measured skin temperature on the hands and feet of people as they entered a relaxed state. Sure enough, they could eventually teach themselves to warm their hands and feet on their own by using their minds.

THE MIND AND METABOLISM

After finishing my postdoctoral fellowship, I joined the faculty of Harvard Medical School in 1974 and began to experiment with relaxation techniques as well as biofeedback. In one of the studies at Harvard, we showed that relaxation is as good as biofeedback at lowering blood pressure.

In 1977, Duke University recruited me to head its new biofeedback program. I moved from Boston to the South, but continued the same research focus, examining numerous mind-body therapies and their effects on migraine headaches, blood pressure, and Raynaud's disease.

As director of the biofeedback lab, I was being asked constantly to consult on the use of biofeedback to help patients with all sorts of problems at Duke Hospital. Most of these patients had migraine headaches, hypertension, or Raynaud's disease. A year after I arrived at Duke, I bumped into a young endocrinologist, Mark Feinglos, M.D., who asked me to see a patient who had diabetes. This prompted me to study how the mind influences metabolism and diabetes, about which I knew very little at the time.

During our first meeting, Mark told me about several of his patients whose diabetes could not be completely controlled with medication. Suspecting they were under significant stress and that the stress was somehow contributing to the diabetes, he asked whether I could work with one patient to see if mind-body techniques could lower her blood sugar. At first, I was skeptical. Could the brain really control metabolism?

"Do you think you can help her?" he asked.

"I have no idea," was my honest reply. As Mark explained how he thought mind-body therapies might help his patients, I became more and more convinced and more excited to give it a try.

Mark explained that relaxation training could lower levels of stress hormones, something I already knew from my work with heart disease and Raynaud's. Then he went on to tell me something I didn't know: that stress hormones such as cortisol and epinephrine influence blood sugar. Increases in these hormones can elevate blood sugar. It made sense that lowering those hormones would, in turn, lower blood sugar.

In a stressful or dangerous situation, the body produces stress hormones that help you escape danger or fight it. This *fight-or-flight response* starts in your brain as soon as you mentally recognize a threat, whether it's your boss breathing down your neck or your child crying with a high fever. When you become anxious, stressed, or angry, nerve cells in the part of your brain called the hypothalamus send messages to your nearby pituitary gland, which sends messages to your adrenal glands (located above your kidneys) to release the stress hormones adrenaline and cortisol, among others. These hormones tell blood vessels in your muscles to dilate and blood vessels in your skin, kidneys, and intestines to constrict.

During fight or flight, blood pressure, heart rate, breathing rate, muscle tension, and blood flow to the muscles all increase. Stomach and intestinal activity slows, and blood sugar is released from the liver and muscle stores, readying a supply of energy for the body to use to run or fend off an attacker. Certain stress hormones also make available other stored energy, such as fatty acids, for the body to burn for fight or flight. For people who do not have diabetes, this is adaptive; their pancreas correctly recognizes a rise in blood sugar and responds by secreting the hormone insulin, which helps shuttle sugar into the cells that need it. For people with diabetes, however, this creates a potential problem. Because of their inability to produce enough insulin or use the insulin they have, their blood sugar goes up and does not come down. Either insulin doesn't let blood sugar into their cells, or their pancreas doesn't secrete enough insulin to let enough blood sugar into their cells. Stress hormones can also suppress the pancreas's ability to secrete insulin. The hormones released during fight or flight therefore have a double effect: creating high blood sugar and hampering the body's ability to get that sugar where it belongs.

There are many stress hormones, but four are the most important ones for people with diabetes:

- CORTISOL. This hormone primarily acts as an anti-inflammatory in the body, helping to ease tissue inflammation. It also stimulates the liver to convert stored carbohydrate and protein into glucose (or blood sugar) and release it into the blood. It is secreted by the outer layer of the adrenal gland, called the adrenal cortex.

- EPINEPHRINE. This hormone stimulates the conversion of glycogen (a starch stored in the liver) to sugar. It also stimulates the release of free fatty acids from fat cells. The more free fatty acids in the blood, the less sugar the cells need. Epinephrine can also prevent the pancreas from releasing insulin. It is secreted by the inside of the adrenal gland called the adrenal medulla.

- NOREPINEPHRINE. Norepinephrine is a neurotransmitter (chemical messenger) that is chemically very similar to epinephrine. Norepinephrine is secreted by nerves in the sympathetic nervous system from one nerve to another and can impair insulin secretion.

- GROWTH HORMONE. Growth hormone can mobilize energy reserves and limit the effects of insulin on the ability of muscle to use blood sugar. This hormone is secreted by the pituitary gland.

These hormones are beneficial during athletic competition and periods of mental or psychological stress. At these times, you want your body to release as much stored sugar as possible so that your muscles, heart, and brain have sufficient energy to deal with the crisis. Assuming you don't have diabetes, your muscles will burn that sugar for energy, and your blood sugar level barely rises.

When you have diabetes, because of a lack of insulin or the inability to respond to it (insulin resistance), your muscles and other tissues can't get that sugar, which remains high in the blood. To complicate matters, certain stress hormones such as cortisol and epinephrine may also contribute to insulin resistance in people predisposed to diabetes.

When you are under chronic stress that lasts day after day—

such as going through a divorce or experiencing difficulties at work—your body reacts with the fight-or-flight response. Over a long period of time, the effects of stress can be profound for those with diabetes and for those without it. Chronically elevated epinephrine and cortisol can raise your blood pressure, spike your blood lipids, suppress your immunity, and even cause bone loss. Recent research has also suggested that chronically elevated stress hormones can impair brain function. These hormones have also been linked with many diseases, including migraine headaches, irritable bowel syndrome, and even obesity (cortisol promotes the buildup of body fat).

Just as your brain can set off the fight-or-flight response, it can also reverse the effect. The hypothalamus, a small area at the base of the brain, controls the autonomic nervous system. Part of this system is the sympathetic nervous system, which regulates arousal and fight or flight, but the parasympathetic system counters the fight-or-flight response by producing the opposite effects. The parasympathetic nervous system can slow heart rate, decrease blood pressure, and increase insulin secretion. As David Shapiro, Herb Benson, and others have shown, the thinking part of the brain can be taught to control the hypothalamus.

Mark finished explaining how mental relaxation might work to control blood sugar and metabolism. It seemed plausible to me that by decreasing the activity of the sympathetic nervous system, activating the parasympathetic nervous system, and decreasing the release of cortisol from the adrenal glands, relaxation techniques would turn off the fight-or-flight response and could lower blood sugar.

THE BRAIN AND BLOOD SUGAR

Although the physiology made sense, the notion that people could be trained to lower their blood sugar was a radical concept in the late 1970s. At that time, no one was looking at how to use the mind to influence blood sugar control, but we had some historical support for our hunch.

Stress is a major disruption of health. Even in the 1970s,

when this was not as accepted as it is today, Mark and I could refer to some medical history that was specific to stress, poor health, and blood sugar. For instance, Hippocrates, the fourth-century B.C. founder of Western medicine, linked health with a proper balance of mind, body, and environment. In the second century, Galen, a Greek doctor, noted that women who were depressed tended to be at risk for breast cancer. In the mid-1800s, Claude Bernard, a French physiologist, linked the internal state of the brain to the proper function of the body, describing the brain's main function as maintaining a state of homeostasis, or balance, in the body. Theoretically, external forces such as stress could be responsible for some diseases.

Bernard, now considered the father of modern physiology, was one of the earliest researchers to show that the brain can control blood sugar levels. He also observed a link between stress and diabetes. Bernard produced abnormally high blood sugar levels in normal rabbits simply by stimulating an area of their hypothalamus with a thin skewer-like device. When he poked this particular area of the brain, blood sugar increased. Bernard hypothesized that the brain was the control center of the metabolism that led to diabetes.

Later in the 1800s, Henry Maudsley, one of the founders of modern psychiatry, noted that diabetes often followed sudden trauma. He reported the story of a military officer, who, upon discovering that his wife was having an affair, immediately developed the disease. In the 1890s, William Osler, possibly the most famous modern physician, suggested that stress probably plays a role in type 2 diabetes. He routinely prescribed rest and opiates, drugs that produce relaxation, for his diabetes patients. Walter Cannon, a scientist at Harvard during the 1940s who coined the term *fight-or-flight response,* found that cats' blood sugar rose when they were frightened or stressed.

Yet after the discovery of insulin in the 1920s, researchers largely abandoned the notion that the brain might be involved in diabetes. Instead, they focused on the pancreas as its ultimate cause. Scientists have long thought that a defect in the cells of the pancreas makes it unable to recognize high blood sugar levels and respond with adequate insulin. In type 1 diabetes, destruction of the pancreas by the body's immune system is known to cause the disease, but the role of the pancreas in type 2 diabetes was less clear.

The pancreas certainly plays a role in diabetes, but it's not the control center of all metabolic processes. The brain is. Pancreatic cells can sense a rise in blood sugar, but the brain can also influence insulin release through the release of stress hormones and nerve stimulation.

How might the brain be involved in type 2 diabetes? Mark and I suspected that people with diabetes have different levels of certain chemical messengers in the brain than do those without the disease. Brain function depends on chemicals released by nerve cells in the brain which stimulate or inhibit other nerves. We've since learned that different neurotransmitters interact with each other in complex ways. Some are responsible for feelings of calmness and euphoria and others for feelings of anger and frustration. You've probably heard about one of them in particular: serotonin.

Low levels of serotonin have been implicated in depression, hostility, and obesity. If you have diabetes, low levels of serotonin may cause you to respond to stress more, thereby elevating your levels of stress hormones. In other words, it may cause your fight-or-flight response to kick in more quickly than someone else's.

Raising levels of serotonin in both animals and people causes them to eat less and lose weight. This brain chemical also plays a role in satiety, so low levels may cause you to overeat and gain weight, which in turn makes your cells resistant to insulin. Mark and I didn't know all of this back in the 1970s, but we knew enough to know that we wanted to know more.

A SIGNIFICANT CASE

It seemed worth trying to answer the question: Does blood sugar rise and fall automatically, or could we use the mind-body connection to alter the reaction? One of Mark's sickest patients, Janice, in Duke Hospital would help us find out. Her uncontrollable blood sugar threatened to make her blind.

The Janice I met in the fall of 1978 was small, frail, and scared. She was only in her early thirties, but insulin and diet had failed to bring down her dangerously high blood sugar levels. As a result, the blood vessels in her eyes were wearing away and bleeding. She was losing her eyesight. Janice was also under a lot of stress. The fear of losing her eyesight was creating stress. She was caught in a vicious cycle.

I spent a week teaching Janice to relax by using a method called progressive muscle relaxation. The technique involves systematically tensing and relaxing different muscles in the body to achieve a state of deep relaxation. In addition to the relaxation exercises, I attached sensors to Janice's muscles that connected to an electromyography biofeedback machine. As Janice tried to relax, the machine gave her feedback in the form of various pitched tones that let her know whether she was truly reducing her muscle tension.

Janice caught on quickly and soon did not need the machine to tell her when she was relaxed and when she was tense. More important, Janice's blood sugar began to normalize. After several weeks, her eye condition started to improve, and she was discharged from the hospital. She didn't lose her vision, which just days before had seemed a certainty.

Janice's recovery was so dramatic that Mark and I excitedly began talking about its possible implications for diabetes treatment. We were filled with questions. Was Janice an anomaly, or would the technique work on others too? Could it help people with diabetes who didn't seem to suffer from excess stress? Why did this relaxation technique work? Although we knew that it probably helped lower stress hormones, we weren't convinced that was the reason.

Janice's remarkable recovery has led me on a lifelong mission to uncover the psychological aspects of blood sugar control. At the time, no one else was working in this area, but the physiological logic and Janice's startling recovery were enough to encourage me to forge ahead even if no one else seemed convinced that I was on to something.

At times, I felt like a detective trying to solve a murder mystery. Diabetes eventually kills people by weakening their heart, kidneys, and other organs, but in the 1970s, we didn't know why. We knew that people with diabetes had high levels of sugar in their blood, but we didn't know what caused those levels to remain high. We thought that the mind played some sort of a role but didn't know what.

In the many decades since treating Janice, I have learned that stress does indeed raise blood sugar levels. Even in people who don't have diabetes but may be prone to develop it eventually, psychological factors may work to lower insulin secretion and raise blood sugar.

3

The First Blood Sugar Booster

Stress May Trigger and Aggravate Diabetes

SINCE that first experience with Janice, I've learned that using a biofeedback machine isn't necessary to lower blood sugar. Progressive muscle relaxation alone can help. I've taught progressive muscle relaxation to hundreds of people with diabetes. One of my patients was a minister whose blood sugar level was twice as high on Sundays, when he faced the stress of preaching, as during the rest of the week. Besides the stage fright associated with preaching to a large congregation, he also had the stress of working with a large congregation—listening to them and comforting them, and dealing with parish, staff, and lay politics and conflicts. Clergy are never off-duty, and their personal ethics, decisions, and actions are held to the highest standards by those around them. To make matters worse for this minister, he had an obsessive personality type, so his thought processes magnified his stress. Sermons, in particular, were a big deal for him. He wasn't so much scared to talk in public, but he very much wanted to get his message across to everyone in the congregation.

I taught him the same relaxation technique that I had taught to Janice, but this time combined it with something called systematic desensitization, that is, systematically using progressive muscle relaxation to lower your stress response in a stressful situation. In our first session, the minister used the relaxation technique to calm down; once he was relaxed, I asked him to imagine giving a sermon. As soon as he noticed his heartbeat speeding, his hands sweating, or other signs of stress, he would use the relaxation technique to calm down, taking his attention away from the imaginary sermon and back to relaxing his muscles. When he had calmed down again, he again imagined giving a sermon. Eventually, he was able to preach with a calm mind and body, and his blood sugar levels remained under control on Sundays.

Here's another example. For twelve years, Mrs. Jones, another of Mark's patients, kept her diabetes under control with exercise and oral medications. But she began having frequent episodes of high blood sugar, although she was still seemingly doing everything right. During her physical, Mark asked whether her lifestyle had changed recently. It had. She'd taken on new responsibilities at work, and her job was more stressful. She felt anxious during the day and had trouble falling asleep at night. Mark suggested that the stress might be causing the high blood sugar levels. Mrs. Jones spoke to her boss, who lightened her workload. As she felt more relaxed on the job over the next few weeks, her diabetes improved.

Even good stress or excitement can raise blood sugar. One of my colleagues who has diabetes noticed that his blood sugar shot up whenever he attended a Duke University basketball game. The excitement from cheering on the Blue Devils, the Duke basketball team, mobilizes sugar in the same way that a traffic jam would, so he learned that he must take some extra insulin before entering the stadium in order to keep his blood sugar levels in check.

Riding a roller coaster will raise blood sugar in most people, and sex probably does as well. No one wants to avoid the pleasure of excitement, and it's not necessarily desirable to try to remain relaxed when in the middle of a basketball game or the heat of passion. Understanding that even good stress can raise blood sugar can help you to time your medication doses better.

PUTTING STRESS TO THE TEST

As a scientist, I knew Janice's recovery could be dismissed as merely anecdotal, so I decided to do a case control study—albeit a small one. Mark and I asked twelve patients with type 2 diabetes to stay at the Duke University Hospital for nine days. They stayed in regular hospital rooms in a long hallway that looked much like a dormitory setting, not the most exciting place to spend a week of your life. We asked six of the patients to do nothing other than eat, sleep, and watch television. In other words, they took a time-out from their normal lives. The other six had the same orders, except that we taught them the progressive muscle relaxation technique that I had taught Janice.

We tested each patient's glucose tolerance at the beginning of the week and at the week's end. After nine days, the patients who had learned how to relax had improved glucose tolerance, and their blood sugar levels were lower than those who didn't learn to relax.

That study left me wondering why it worked. Blood samples from these patients revealed that the ones who had practiced relaxation had lower levels of the stress hormone cortisol than those who did not. Thus, cortisol seemed to be one player in the stress–blood sugar connection. Although relaxation appeared to work by lowering cortisol, this did not necessarily tell us how stress could raise blood sugar or if stress could contribute to the onset of diabetes.

Sometimes in life, you're blessed by meeting the right person at the right time. For me, that chance opportunity came in the form of a medical student named Elizabeth Livingston (who is now a gynecologist at Duke). Elizabeth had studied at Harvard as an undergraduate and had worked in a lab with *ob/ob* mice, a strain that had been bred to gain weight spontaneously and develop diabetes. Study results on these mice often conflicted. In some studies, the *ob/ob* mice had very high blood sugar levels. In others, their blood sugar was normal—under seemingly the same conditions.

Elizabeth and I began talking about my experiments with stress, diabetes, and relaxation, and she had a light-bulb moment. She told me that at Harvard Medical School, the *ob/ob* mice that developed high blood sugar were housed in a different lab from the ones that had normal blood sugar levels. Though both sets of mice ate the same food, had the same genetics, and underwent the same experiments, their living conditions were quite different. In one lab, the mice were housed with rats, a natural enemy. It was akin to housing humans with lions or birds with cats. Elizabeth wondered whether the stress from living with rats was causing that set of *ob/ob* mice to develop diabetes.

We decided to find out. We obtained some *ob/ob* mice and housed them in our labs. We first measured their blood sugar in an undisturbed state. Then we placed each mouse into a mild stressful situation that would have a psychological effect on them but would not harm them. We put each mouse in a little wire mesh envelope that restrained their movement. Just as you might feel if you were in a straitjacket, the mesh envelope annoyed but did not harm the mice. Their blood sugar shot sky high—into the diabetic range—compared to *ob/ob* mice that were not placed in the restraining device. They also had reduced insulin secretion.

We wanted to see if other types of stress would produce the same results and also wanted to see if the unique genetics of the *ob/ob* mice made them prone to stress-induced rises in blood sugar. So we got a set of *ob/ob* mice along with a set of their nondiabetic cousins, called B6 mice, which were identical to the *ob/ob* mice except for one mutant gene unique to the *ob/ob*. We put both strains of mice on a moving platform, which created an earthquake-type situation. As with the wire mesh envelope, this was a mild stressor that was annoying but caused no harm.

The *ob/ob* mice had slightly higher blood sugar levels than their lean B6 cousins to start with, but those levels skyrocketed when we placed them on the moving platform. In contrast, the lean B6 mice had a much smaller rise in blood sugar and got used to the shaking platform. After a number of sessions, they eventually didn't respond with a rise in blood sugar when we placed them on the platform. The *ob/ob* mouse, however, never got used to the situation and always responded with high blood sugar.

That taught us that physical stress could spike blood sugar levels in all mice, but especially in genetically susceptible ones. We began to wonder whether some mice were genetically more stress responsive than others and whether mental stress would produce the same results.

To create "mental" stress in the mice, we used classical conditioning, a technique developed by Pavlov in the early 1900s. We sounded a metronome for several minutes before placing the mice on the moving platform, repeating this procedure multiple times. Just as Pavlov's dogs salivated upon hearing a bell that they associated with food, the *ob/ob* mice, but not the B6 mice, eventually responded to the sound of the metronome with high blood sugar as soon as the ticking began, before we ever moved the platform. This told us that "mental" or anticipated stress could raise blood sugar just as high as physical stress. We now knew that stress could be very subtle. You didn't have to be running for your life for stress to affect your glucose.

Next, we wanted to see if we could create a similar result from "social stress" in mice. The late physiologist James Henry had shown that he could raise mice's blood pressure by housing them in a large group situation where each was forced to interact with many others in order to share food, water, and mates. We tried the same thing with *ob/ob* mice and B6 mice. Sure enough, after several weeks in the group housing situation, the blood sugar of the *ob/ob* mice rose to diabetic levels, while that of the B6 remained normal. We had proved that social stress could trigger diabetes in genetically predisposed animals.

But we had one last question to answer: Why? We suspected that stress hormones were at work, but we wanted to know for sure.

In a number of experiments, we tested how activating and then deactivating the sympathetic nervous system (the one involved in fight or flight) affected blood sugar. When we injected mice with the stress hormone epinephrine, their blood sugar went up. In a different experiment, we gave the mice tranquilizers, which shut down the sympathetic nervous system, before placing them in the restraining device. The tranquilized mice did not respond with high sugar; the nontranquilized mice did.

With each experiment, we became more and more convinced that stress and type 2 diabetes were intricately linked, particularly in people who are genetically prone to the disease. We began to suspect that the same subset of genes that make one person prone to diabetes also make that person respond differently to stress.

As we studied the *ob/ob* mice, we found that even the lean B6 mouse, in contrast to other strains of mice, responded to stress with increased levels of blood sugar. Of course, their sugar didn't go up as much as that of the *ob/ob,* but it still increased. We wondered whether the *ob/ob* mouse was diabetic because it had a gene that made it fat (no matter what it ate) and whether the B6 also carried genes for diabetes but was not diabetic because it wasn't fat. Since mouse food is typically very low in fat (about 4 percent), we wondered what would happen to B6 mice if they ate a diet similar to that of humans. To test our theory, we fed B6 mice as well as other types of mice a diet high in fat. Sure enough, the B6 mice gained weight and developed full-blown diabetes, whereas the other mice did not.

This result suggested that an increase in blood sugar in response to stress was a marker for individuals predisposed to diabetes. To test that theory fully, we needed to study a group of humans who, like the B6 mice, were genetically prone to develop diabetes. Because the Pima Indians in Arizona are perhaps the most afflicted with diabetes, we decided to find out if they were also stress responsive. We tested a group of young Pimas who had not yet developed diabetes, as well as a group of Caucasians the same age from the Phoenix area.

We gave both groups a mental arithmetic task that required they perform multiplication in their heads at a rapid pace. This task is a common laboratory stress that is known to raise epinephrine levels and cause changes in blood pressure and heart rate. During the test, the Pimas' blood sugar went up, but the

Caucasians' blood sugar went down. It wasn't that the Pimas found the test harder or more stressful than the Caucasians. Both responded to the test with a similar rise in heart rate. The Pimas were simply predisposed to respond to stress with high blood sugar.

THE EVOLUTION OF STRESS

Because stress contributes to diabetes and the rates of diabetes are at their highest ever, you may wonder whether humans are more stressed now than they were 100, 200, 300, or even 1,000 years ago.

In my opinion, no. People have always been subjected to stress, whether the stress of trying to find the next meal or the stress of trying to get to work on time. My grandmother raised four children as a widow during the Great Depression. Was her life any less stressful than what a single mother faces today? I don't think so.

What is different is the rest of our lifestyle. One hundred years ago, rates of diabetes were much lower because few of us could find enough calories to overeat, particularly fat calories. Also, we were physically more active. Cars, drive-through restaurants, Internet shopping, and other modern conveniences have nearly eliminated our need to move, which has contributed greatly to diabetes.

CONVINCING EVIDENCE

The research on stress includes such a wealth of evidence that it's hard to find a scientist who doesn't believe that stress contributes to high blood sugar in diabetes. The famous physiologist Hans Selye, who coined the term *stress,* differentiated between noxious stress, which he termed *distress,* and the stress of excitement, which he termed *eustress.* We researchers now know that there's not much of a difference between eustress and distress: the body reacts in the same manner in response to both. Although you don't necessarily want to immunize yourself from eustress, you do need to learn how to recognize all types of stress that will raise your blood sugar and find a remedy.

In people who are already predisposed to develop diabetes because of their genetic makeup, stress can bring on the first symptoms and cause the first diagnosis. In someone with type 1 diabetes, where the immune system mistakenly destroys beta cells of the pancreas, stress increases the body's demand for insulin, which speeds the appearance of the disease. Since the person doesn't have enough beta cells, the body can't produce enough insulin. The demands of stress overwhelm the body's ability to make insulin, and symptoms of diabetes begin to appear. The same may be true for type 2 diabetes. For someone already close to exhibiting symptoms, stress may bring them on faster by lowering insulin levels, raising blood sugar levels, raising insulin levels, or making cells more resistant to insulin.

In people with type 1 or type 2, stress may make the difference between getting blood sugar levels under control or not. In Chapter 6, you'll learn how to find out if you are stress responsive, and in Chapter 7, you'll find out what to do about it.

4

The Second Blood Sugar Booster

Diabetes Control and Depression Seem Closely Linked

PEOPLE with diabetes are more prone to depression and obesity, people with depression are more prone to diabetes and obesity, and people with obesity are more prone to diabetes and depression. People who are depressed tend to eat more and exercise less, lifestyle factors that contribute to obesity. People who are obese tend to have cells that are resistant to the effects of insulin, which leads to diabetes and further overeating. All of these traits are linked.

As my research into stress and diabetes began to build back in the 1980s, Dr. Bernard Carroll, then chairman of the Department of Psychiatry at Duke, mentioned to me that he thought depression might also be linked to diabetes. His patients who suffered from severe depression often had chronic elevations in the stress hormone cortisol, which plays a critical role in elevating blood sugar.

Dr. Carroll often discovered undiagnosed diabetes in his depressed patients. He also had found mild elevations in blood sugar even in nondiabetic people with depression. Depression, he noted, makes the body resistant to the hormone insulin. I was intrigued and decided to see if others had noticed the same connection. After carefully examining the medical literature, I found that many physicians who treated people with diabetes had noticed the link between the two conditions long before researchers had. For instance, in the early 1980s, there were case reports of patients going into remission from both depression and diabetes symptoms after shock therapy. A few researchers even reported that shock therapy could improve blood sugar in diabetic mice.

We scientists at Duke and elsewhere began to investigate depression in patients with diabetes. We found depression tougher to study than stress, however. One problem was that physicians usually prescribe antidepressants to people with any chronic illness. Any illness that limits activity, restricts diet, or produces serious physical complications can produce depression. Though it's a blessing that people now commonly receive treatment for their depression, it's now hard to find study subjects with diabetes who aren't already taking antidepressants, which makes it difficult to perform controlled studies.

A DEPRESSED MIND

Many people casually refer to themselves as depressed. "I'm so depressed today," someone might say. They say, "I can't stand when it rains" or "The news really depresses me." True depression is not the same thing as temporary sadness. True depression lasts more than a few hours or a day or two. It interferes with the ability to function and maintain interest in life for weeks on end.

The medical community defines depression as feeling sad and having diminished interest in nearly all activities most of the day or most days. Along with this persistent sadness or disinterest, a person with depression may have many of the following symptoms:

- A significant increase or decrease in weight or appetite
- Feelings of worthlessness, hopelessness, or guilt
- Sleep disturbances
- Lack of sexual desire
- Fatigue
- Poor concentration
- Slowed or fuzzy thinking

- Indecision
- Moodiness
- Recurrent thoughts about death or suicide

About 18 million people in the United States are considered depressed. Although scientists don't know precisely what causes depression, the most popular theory centers on abnormal brain chemistry, which may be genetically inherited or triggered by severe stress, grief, or personal loss—or all of these. Depression is much more than a mental illness, however. It seems to drag the entire human body down with it, raising the risk for heart disease, osteoporosis, and cancer. Indeed, depression has been linked with poor health, including diabetes, for four centuries.

THE DEPRESSION-DIABETES CONNECTION

Scientists are not completely sure about how or why depression and diabetes are connected, but we know that the connection exists. Statistics show this clearly. Diabetes more than doubles the odds of suffering from depression at some point. One-third of people with diabetes have been diagnosed with significant depression and 11 percent with major depression—twice the rate of depression in the nondiabetic population.

What comes first: depression or diabetes? Some scientists argue that the lifestyle changes and the health threat associated with diabetes are enough to make anyone feel depressed. Perhaps you remember feeling deflated after you learned about your diabetes diagnosis. Suddenly you had to alter much of your life. You were told to watch your diet, begin an exercise program, lose weight, and monitor your blood sugar numerous times each day. You may have felt even more deflated and anxious when you learned about the possible complications of your disease—heart attack, stroke, blindness, nerve disease, and kidney failure.

There's some research to support the idea that a diagnosis of a chronic illness can trigger depression. For example, one study published in *Diabetes Care* found that the more severe and time-consuming the treatment regimen, the more likely it is that a patient will become depressed. Some scientists who believe that diabetes itself triggers depression also argue that high blood sugar causes biochemical changes in the brain that can lead to depression. Again, some research supports this notion.

Some of the association between diabetes and depression may certainly be due to the burden of having a chronic disease, but research shows that people with diabetes are even more prone to depression than people suffering from other chronic diseases, such as arthritis. Reduced functioning, social isolation, financial hardship, unemployment, and other problems crop up in all chronic illnesses. Yet cardiac rehabilitation patients with diabetes are twice as likely to become depressed as cardiac rehab patients without diabetes.

Depression is common even in people with diabetes who have not yet developed complications. Statistics tell us that in the vast majority of cases, the depression came first and the diabetes came second—for example:

- Japanese researchers tested 2,764 people for depression and then tracked their health for eight years. Those diagnosed with depression at the beginning of the study were two times as likely to develop diabetes during the following eight years. The researchers published their results in *Diabetes Care* in 2000.
- A Johns Hopkins University thirteen-year-long study of about 2,000 people, published in *Diabetes Care* in 1996, found that those who were diagnosed with depression were more than twice as likely to develop diabetes.
- A Kaiser Permanente's Center for Health Research study found that people with diabetes were more likely to have been treated for depression six months before their diabetes diagnosis compared to those without diabetes.

Though it is interesting to speculate on whether depression causes diabetes or vice versa, *the more important question for you as an individual is whether depression worsens your diabetes.* The answer to that question is complicated.

When I first became interested in the question of how depression affects diabetes, there had already been many different scientific studies on the topic, some of which showed that depression made diabetes worse; others did not. As I attempted to explain this confusion, I noticed that most of the research on diabetes and depression combined patients with type 1 diabetes with those with type 2 diabetes. This made no sense to me because type 1 and type 2 diabetes are completely different diseases. So in a study we completed at Duke just a few years ago, we asked more than sixty diabetes patients—thirty with type 1 and thirty-four with type 2—a series of questions to assess their mood and determine if they had depression. We also measured the hemoglobin AC1, which gives us average blood sugar levels over a period of twelve to sixteen weeks.

At the end of the study, when we compared blood sugar levels to those who scored high on our depression questionnaire, we uncovered a strong relationship between those with type 1 diabetes and depression and poor blood sugar control. In those with type 2 and depression, however, we didn't find any connection with poor blood sugar control. Several other studies that all support our findings have since considered people with type 1 and type 2 separately. For instance, a thirty-six-week study of people with type 1 diabetes found that blood sugar fluctuations mirrored the fluctuations of depressive symptoms. Depression dropped when blood sugar dropped and increased when blood sugar increased.

Does this mean that the connection between depression and diabetes holds true only for those with type 1? At this point we can't say. Because it is often more difficult to control type 1 diabetes than type 2 (people with type 1 diabetes have no insulin), it is likely that the effects of depression will be more pronounced in those with type 1 diabetes.

HOW DEPRESSION INFLUENCES BLOOD SUGAR

Depression can influence diabetes in three different ways. First, depression can raise the level of stress hormones, which can raise blood sugar directly. Second, depression can raise blood sugar indirectly by hindering how you take care of your-self. People who are depressed are less likely to exercise, eat right, take their medication, and test their blood sugar. Third, abnormal levels of certain brain chemicals may predispose certain people to both depression and diabetes.

Let's start with the stress hormone levels. A depressed brain sends out signals that it needs more sugar, which mobilizes the stress hormone cortisol, among others. People with depression have higher overall levels of cortisol twenty-four hours a day than those who are not depressed.

Because stress hormones such as cortisol and epinephrine stimulate the liver to release sugar into the blood, hinder the pancreas from releasing insulin, and block insulin's ability to shuttle sugar into cells, it makes sense that higher levels of these stress hormones may trigger or aggravate diabetes in people genetically prone to the condition. In people who are at risk for developing diabetes and already are insulin resistant, higher stress hormone levels may increase the demand for insulin, tax the pancreas, and lead to full-blown diabetes. In someone who already has been diagnosed with diabetes, depression may prevent lifestyle changes and medication from keeping blood sugar under control.

Depressive symptoms such as fatigue, memory problems, lack of concentration, inactivity, and appetite changes interfere with how you take care of yourself. When you feel tired, you don't feel like exercising or cooking a healthy meal. When you can't think clearly, you can't remember the last time you tested your blood sugar or if you've taken your medication. When you feel hungry, you tend to overeat. In a study of fifty outpatients who had type 1 diabetes, depressive symptoms made patients less likely to visit their doctors, follow a healthy diet, and exercise. Other studies have found similar results. One found that those with depression are more likely to drop out of weight-control programs.

When self-care deteriorates, blood sugar control does too! This may explain why depression seems to worsen type 1 diabetes more than type 2. When self-care lapses in someone with type 1 diabetes, blood sugar rises quickly, but it does not shoot up as quickly in someone with type 2. With more research, we may better be able to explain the discrepancy.

Another theory about why both depression and diabetes occur together centers on levels of brain chemicals called neurotransmitters. We researchers have little proof, but we suspect that people who are prone to depression and diabetes have different levels of certain brain chemicals—or possibly a different brain structure—from those not prone to either illness.

Science is still uncovering the roles of these chemicals. It has revealed that particular brain chemicals control emotions and memories, as well as basic instincts such as hunger, pleasure, and sexual arousal. Several neurotransmitters, called the biogenic amines, have been associated with depression, hunger, and glucose metabolism. These include norepinephrine, serotonin, and histamine. Neurons (or nerve cells) in your brain communicate with one another by secreting tiny quantities of these chemicals. When a particular type of nerve cell becomes activated, it releases one or more of these biogenic amines, which then influence many other cells.

In the 1960s, Dr. Joseph Schildkraut at Harvard Medical School came up with the theory that depression results from a lack of norepinephrine. He was able to show that drugs that increase the concentration of norepinephrine and serotonin can lift the mood of severely depressed patients.

Early antidepressants such as Tofranil (imipramine), Elavil (amitriptyline), and Sinequan (doxepin), which worked on several different biogenic amines at once, did indeed help lift depression. They also made people hungry and induced considerable weight gain. In fact, Dr. Patrick Lustman at Washington University showed that while many drugs that treat depression generally improve diabetes, some of the early antidepressants actually made blood sugar control worse.

Because of these problems and the fact that overdoses of these drugs could be lethal (a real problem when administering them to depressed and possibly suicidal patients), the drug manufacturer Eli Lilly developed Prozac, a medication that specifically targets serotonin receptors. This medication, called a selective serotonin reuptake inhibitor (SSRI), did not affect norepinephrine or histamine and therefore did not have many of the side effects of the earlier drugs.

Some scientists believe that the same deficiency in serotonin that triggers depression may also somehow trigger diabetes. SSRIs are thought to lift depression primarily by enhancing the activity and concentration of serotonin in the brain. Indeed, drugs such as Prozac, which increase serotonin levels, also tend to improve blood sugar control. Enhancing serotonin may reduce hunger and speed up metabolism. Some weight-loss drugs, like fenfluramine (Pondimin) or dexfenfluramine (Redux), which cause nerve cells to release serotonin, were also thought to work this way, but they turned out to have serious side effects and were eventually taken off the market.

RISKY BUSINESS

Whatever the cause and no matter which comes first, depression sharply raises the risk of diabetic complications. Several studies have shown that women with diabetes develop heart disease much faster if they are also depressed.

Depression alters more than just diabetes. Like stress, depression also raises the risk for just about everything, making it a whole-body condition. Depression complicates many disorders, such as heart disease, cancer, osteoporosis, and pain syndromes. It may also trigger them. Here are some examples:

- If you are depressed when you have a heart attack, your ability to recover is greatly reduced. A 1993 study published in the *Journal of the American Medical Association* found that depressed patients who had suffered a heart attack tended to die earlier than those who were not depressed.
- Depression may adversely affect the blood clotting system. During fight or flight, sticky cells called platelets increase in number in an attempt to clot blood should you get cut. Too many platelets can cause heart attacks and strokes. Research shows that depressed patients have a higher blood clotting activation than those who are not depressed.

- People who are depressed tend to develop osteoporosis. Some researchers have equated depression with smoking and genetics as a risk factor for the bone loss disease. Again, cortisol may be to blame.
- Though scientists still aren't sure which comes first, depression is highly correlated with cancer, with 23 to 60 percent of cancer patients also having depression. Cancer may make many people depressed, but for some, it might be the other way around.
- Depression somehow alters the immune system, creating unusually high levels of disease fighters called cytokines, which may compromise immunity and let cancerous cells multiply unchecked.

WHAT YOU CAN DO FOR YOUR DEPRESSION

Now that you know about the connection between diabetes and depression, the most important question remains: Can you do anything about it? The answer to that question is a strong yes. Though depression is largely thought to be a biochemical problem in the brain, a wealth of research shows that you don't necessarily need to take antidepressants to get depression—and blood sugar—under control.

A series of studies done by Dr. Patrick Lustman and colleagues at the Washington University School of Medicine in St. Louis have found that depression treatment—through the use of antidepressants or behavioral therapy—helped get blood sugar under control. One study in particular looked at how cognitive behavior therapy could help lift depression and improve blood sugar. Among all the methods, including medication, cognitive behavior therapy resulted in the highest success rate for relieving depression: 85 percent. This type of therapy teaches you to identify self-defeating thoughts, examine them, and replace them with positive thoughts. It's one of the techniques of the Mind-Body Diabetes Revolution program and is presented in Chapter 8.

The benefits that come from cognitive behavior therapy are enormous. You will notice a difference in your mood in as little as ten weeks and in your blood sugar within about six months.

Most important, you'll sharply reduce your risk of diabetic complications. The therapy will also help you to adopt healthy habits, such as eating right and exercising, which both improve your diabetes outlook.

In Chapter 10, you'll learn about a special program that will help you break the depression-obesity-diabetes cycle by helping you tune in to your hunger cues. Combining this program with cognitive behavior therapy will create the one-two punch you need to overcome depression and diabetes—and to help you lose weight.

5

The Final Blood Sugar Booster

How Cynicism, Anger, and Aggression
May Hinder Metabolism

THE link between hostility and poor health may never have been discovered had two cardiologists during the mid-1950s not asked an upholsterer to update the fabric on the chairs in their waiting room. The upholsterer commented to the doctors that each chair displayed an unusual wear pattern: only the front edge of each seat was frayed, whereas the rest of the fabric appeared brand new. The two doctors, Meyer Friedman and Ray Rosenman, began to see that most of their patients seemed to share the same set of personality traits. The cardiologists' patients were hurried, easily angered, hostile, competitive, obsessed about personal achievement, and ambitious—the type of people who would sit on the edge of their seats while waiting for their appointments. This helped explain the cause of the chairs' frayed edges in their waiting room. The doctors also came across a few small studies done by psychiatrists that found that certain personality traits, such as anger, hostility, and aggression, were more common in heart attack patients. Friedman and Rosenman suspected that this set of personality traits might predispose people to develop heart disease. They called people with these traits "type A" and people who didn't have these personality traits "type B."

At first, many researchers and physicians dismissed their theory. Over the years, however, as Friedman, Rosenman, and others performed study after study, many became convinced that type A personality was one of the causes of nearly all diseases. The theory became so popular that the terms have become a part of our everyday language and even people who are not ill refer to themselves as type A or type B.

Since Friedman and Rosenman's studies, researchers have discovered that only certain aspects of type A personality—hostility in particular—put people at risk for poor health. As with people who are prone to stress and depression, hostile personality types may be prone to poor blood sugar control. How and why hostility contributes to poor health is still being researched, but here's the story as we psychologists understand it today.

FROM TYPE A TO HOSTILE

After a series of small, circumstantial studies in the 1960s, Friedman and Rosenman decided to test their theory with a major study of more than 3,000 men. They wanted to see if the men designated as type A at the beginning of the study developed more heart disease than those designated as type B. Eight and a half years later, they got the results they had anticipated: men with type A personalities were twice as likely to develop heart disease as the type Bs. Friedman and Rosenman later did autopsies on patients who had died from heart disease and uncovered more clogged arteries among those who had been designated as type A during their life than those with type B personalities.

These studies created a lot of excitement, and by the 1970s, others had quickly jumped on the type A research wagon. At the time, we at Duke already suspected that stress was somehow related to high blood pressure and many other problems, such as migraine headache and blood sugar control, so it made sense that those with type A personality types would be inherently more stressed than those with the more easygoing type B personalities. More stress meant more stress hormones coursing through their bodies on a regular basis, keeping them in a chronic fight-or-flight mode. Repeatedly throughout the day, as type A personality types argued, rushed, and sweated out each deadline, they also raised their heart rate and blood pressure, shot up their blood sugar, increased their muscle tension, and shut down their intestines. No wonder they were getting heart disease.

In one study we completed during the 1980s, colleagues and I at Duke wanted to see whether type A personality would influence whether stress contributes to diabetes. We selected twenty-one patients with diabetes and used personality questionnaires to test them for type A and type B behavior characteristics. We then tested their blood sugar levels, blood pressure, and heart rate before and after they played a challenging video game for ten minutes. As they played the game, we placed a loud kitchen timer in their field of vision so they knew exactly how many minutes they had left to achieve a maximum score. Halfway through, we told each participant that his or her score was not as high as expected (even if it wasn't true). When we tested blood sugar levels after the game, those with type A personality had much higher blood glucose levels than the type B players, even though both had a similar rise in blood pressure and heart rate.

In a different study at Duke, we asked a teacher to complete a personality questionnaire on twenty-one children with type 1 diabetes. Those children whom the teacher viewed as competitive and hard-driving (components of type A personality) were more likely to show small increases in blood sugar while playing video games. Children seen as easygoing and less competitive (type B personality) tended to show decreases in blood sugar in response to the same task.

Type A, heart disease, and elevated blood sugar levels all seemed to fit together until studies began to conflict. During the mid- and late 1970s, studies found no differences between the health of type A and B personalities. For example, one study followed the health of thousands of patients for several years. At the beginning of the study, patients filled out a questionnaire, the answers to which placed the patients in a type A or type B category. Several years later, when researchers crunched the numbers, they found no difference in heart attack risk among those with type A and those with type B.

At first, some scientists tried to explain away the adverse findings, wondering whether the researchers had correctly identified people as the right personality types. As study after study began to emerge, however, the negative findings began to pile up and became harder to ignore. Rather than allowing the type A theory to die out completely, however, a small group of researchers took a closer look. They began to sort through all of the personality characteristics. Were all of these characteristics bad for health, or just some of them? Was it true, for example, that ambition was bad for one's health? What about competition?

Eventually, after paring away one characteristic after another, two of my colleagues at Duke, Drs. James Blumenthal and Redford Williams, discovered that hostility, a component of the type A personality, was the trait that appeared most related to poor health. Hostility includes characteristics such as cynical mistrust, anger, and aggressive behavior. The other components of the type A pattern, such as impatience, were not related to heart disease.

THE HOSTILE HEART

Redford Williams followed up on his early work with Blumenthal and coined the term *hostility syndrome* to describe a group of risky thoughts and behaviors that include cynicism, anger, and aggression:

• CYNICISM. Hostility starts with the way you think. If you're hostile, you don't trust others and think that most people are selfish and out to get you. You might say things like, "I can never trust others to do the right thing. If I need something done right, I have to do it myself." Such thoughts often lead to anger, the next element of the hostile personality type.

• ANGER. Because of your cynical thoughts, you have a short fuse for your anger. As soon as someone confirms your cynical suspicions—for example, by taking the parking space you were already backing into—the lid for your anger pops off, and you feel irritated, annoyed, and frustrated. This leads to the last element of the hostile personality: aggression.

• Aggression. Your near-constant anger causes you to lash out. You may yell at people, hit them, or shove them. You might displace your anger by kicking the dog or screaming at your kids. You might punch a hole in the wall, tailgate other drivers, or throw objects.

Hostile people are the ones who tailgate you, flash their lights, and make rude hand gestures all within the few seconds you've had to notice that they were behind you in traffic. They're the ones who scream at a cashier at the grocery store because she doesn't know the price of an item. They associate with very few of their neighbors because they believe their neighbors are all out to get them or are talking about them behind their backs.

Physicians have long noticed a connection between a quick temper and heart disease. An English surgeon who lived during the 1700s once said, "My life is in the hands of any rascal who chooses to annoy and tease me." That physician, John Hunter, died—apparently of a heart attack—moments after a heated argument at a hospital board meeting.

Like depression, hostility probably starts with biochemical changes in the brain. In fact, hostility is often associated with depression, and many scientists believe that they may be two facets of the same problem. Williams's work has shown that hostility, like depression, is associated with abnormal serotonin metabolism in the brain. There is also some evidence that drugs useful for depression may help hostile people as well.

Exactly why hostility is associated with increased heart disease is not completely clear. When hostile people think negative thoughts, nerve cells in the hypothalamus send signals to the rest of the body, triggering the same fight-or-flight response seen with stress. Hostile people have elevated cortisol levels, as do people who are chronically depressed. The fight-or-flight response makes the heart beat faster and increases blood pressure. Your arteries in the skin and some organs, such as the kidneys, constrict, and arteries in the muscles open wide. This would all be helpful if the anger were really needed (if you were to follow it up with hand-to-hand combat, for example). But usually you're angry because someone has placed fifteen items on the checkout counter in the ten-items-or-fewer line.

Once triggered, the fight-or-flight response lasts long after the angering situation has passed. This again is part of the body's adaptive nature. If you need to run, it stays triggered to keep up your energy. If you're bleeding, the fight-or-flight response helps clot blood and reduce blood flow to the skin. If you don't need an active fight-or-flight response to run from danger, however, it can erode heart health in a number of ways. First, the rise in blood pressure can damage artery linings. Platelets, the sticky cells in the blood responsible for clotting, clump together more easily and lodge themselves along the sides of arteries that have been damaged by blood pressure. At the same time, fat cells empty their contents, and the liver converts this fat to cholesterol, or blood lipids, which create energy to burn. Even though you are not really running from danger, this excess unused energy can raise blood sugar. Elevated blood lipids could also be responsible for atherosclerosis, or clogged arteries.

Each time you feel hostile, this process could, in theory, slowly increase the degree to which your arteries are clogged. Ultimately, these blockages can become so large that one blocks off an artery entirely. If this occurs in an artery in the heart, a heart attack results. Some studies seem to support this theory. In one study of 1,800 employees who worked for Western Electric, those who scored high on a test of hostility personality traits were more likely to die from heart disease within the following twenty years.

HOSTILITY AND DIABETES

Research about the connection between hostility and heart disease gained momentum during the 1980s and 1990s. At about the same time, another theory about the causes of heart disease became popular.

An endocrinologist and diabetes researcher, Dr. Gerald Reaven, discovered that people who develop heart disease often have a group of abnormalities that look like early diabetes: slightly elevated blood sugar, elevated insulin, obesity (particularly around the gut), and high blood pressure. Many of these people went on to develop diabetes, but others did not. Even those who didn't develop diabetes, however, were prone to developing heart disease. This became known as syndrome X, or metabolic syndrome.

During the late 1990s, a hostility researcher by the name of Ray Niaura decided to see if hostility might be related to syndrome X. His study of 2,280 men found that hostile men were more likely to consume more calories, be overweight, carry most of their excess fat in their abdomen, and have higher triglyceride levels, lower levels of the healthy HDL cholesterol (the type of cholesterol that scoops up excess blood lipids and transports it safely to the liver for disposal), and higher insulin levels. Niaura suggested that hostility affects blood sugar mainly by causing people to eat more and gain weight. Several other investigators found similar results in several studies conducted in Europe.

I was intrigued by these findings and wondered whether the increase in heart disease risk was a result of hostility's effect on stress and blood sugar, which raised risk for heart disease. I was also curious to see whether hostility, like depression, might affect blood sugar through stress hormones. My colleague at Duke, Dr. Williams, was in the middle of a large study to determine the mechanism by which hostility affects heart disease, so I suggested that we collect fasting blood sugar (blood sugar readings taken at least eight hours after a meal) and insulin samples, in addition to the other measures he was planning. We studied ninety-eight men and women and tested their hostility levels and blood sugar, insulin, and other glycemic indicators. No one in this study had diabetes, but many were genetically at risk for developing it.

We found that hostile people tended to have insulin resistance and higher blood sugar levels. In African Americans, this was independent of body weight, which has been blamed in the past for the diabetes-hostility connection. The study seemed to show that hostile people have a genetic short fuse that tends to raise stress hormones more easily and prevent them from being cleared fast enough.

Other research seems to confirm our findings. A May 2003 study published in *Health Psychology*, for example, found that hostile children are more likely to develop metabolic syndrome (obesity, insulin resistance, diabetes, high blood pressure, and high blood cholesterol) than nonhostile children. In a study published in *Diabetes Care* in 2001, investigators studying people from the Virgin Islands found that hostility predicted the onset of diabetes.

A study that looked at other factors of hostility syndrome found that teenage males considered to be aggressive (a component of hostility syndrome) had elevated triglyceride and insulin levels (a precursor to insulin resistance) as well as increased weight three years later compared to teens not designated as aggressive. Another study found that men and women with high anger or hostility scores also had high levels of insulin and blood sugar.

HOSTILITY IS BAD FOR YOUR WHOLE BODY

Hostility does much more than raise the risk for diabetes. When you're prone to anger and lashing out, hostility creates conflict everywhere you go, possibly ruining your marriage and relationships with loved ones, friends, coworkers, supervisors, and clients. Research shows that hostile people tend to have fewer friends and less social support. Hostile people also tend to feel more stress. The more poorly you treat others, the more poorly they treat you. You honk at another driver, and that driver gestures rudely. You yell at your boss; you don't get a raise. It's a vicious cycle. Your hostile behavior makes others do what you fear they will do, which makes you angrier. Treating others badly makes them want to stay away from you, which creates a double problem because research shows that social ties are important to health. People with fewer social ties experience higher death rates.

To counteract stress and unhappiness, hostile personality types tend to self-medicate with alcohol, nicotine, and food, possibly in an unconscious attempt to boost levels of calming brain chemicals. Research shows that hostile people are more likely to smoke, drink, and overeat. One study found that hostile types consume a startling 600 more calories a day than non-hostile types. Hostility may also magnify the stress response, spiking blood pressure, cholesterol, and sugar levels even higher than in a nonhostile person who becomes angry.

WHY YOU'RE HOSTILE

Hostile people share many traits with some types of depressed people. The tendency to develop hostility probably lies in genetics and individual brain chemistry. Hostile people are thought to have similar problems with serotonin and other neurotransmitters as depressed people. If you are hostile, your sympathetic nervous system may be especially touchy. The slightest agitation may set it off, sending stress hormones coursing through your body and making your entire body feel agitated.

In addition to a sensitive fight-or-flight switch, you also may have a sluggish parasympathetic (calming) nervous system. When the parasympathetic nervous system kicks in, it often acts to counter the effects of stress hormones and calm the body. In hostile types, however, the parasympathetic system doesn't kick in as quickly or as strongly, so you're left feeling angry and stressed long after a stressful encounter. Since the parasympathetic nervous system also helps stimulate insulin release, hostility may influence glucose metabolism by working on the pancreas.

In one study, researchers placed an ice pack against the faces of hostile and nonhostile people. The coolness from the ice pack should have activated the calming parasympathetic nervous system. In hostile types, however, the parasympathetic nervous system kicked in for only a couple of minutes, and then the stress hormones returned.

Your touchy sympathetic and sluggish parasympathetic nervous system may be caused by abnormal levels of brain chemicals, particularly serotonin. Some research shows that people with hostility syndrome, like those with depression, have lower levels of serotonin in the brain. Low serotonin may create that short fuse, sending you into fight-or-flight mode earlier and more often. This low serotonin may also explain the tendency of hostile people to self-medicate with nicotine, alcohol, and food. Both nicotine and alcohol dependence have been linked with low levels of serotonin in the brain, and some research shows that drugs that raise serotonin levels can help people quit smoking, recover from alcohol addiction, and lose weight.

Though genetics certainly plays a role in who becomes hostile and who does not, it doesn't tell the whole story. My Duke colleague Dr. Williams, now considered one of the foremost experts on hostility, suspects that genetics can be blamed for only half of the problem. The other half can be blamed on upbringing—on behavior and attitudes you learned. During your childhood, you probably learned some of your thoughts and actions from your parents and others around you. If your parents mistrusted others, they probably passed that mistrust on to you. If your parents reacted to their anger by lashing out, you learned your behavior from them.

We learn to trust others based on our parents' ability to trust us and make us feel secure. Some psychologists suspect that if a child does not learn to trust at least one person within the first two years of life—and that person usually is a parent or caregiver—his or her ability to trust is often impaired later in life.

HOSTILITY AND YOU

Now for the most important question of all: Can you do anything about your hostility? Yes. In one important study, Meyer Friedman, one of the doctors who coined type A, enrolled 1,000 men who had recently suffered a heart attack into a program. He treated two-thirds of them with psychological programs to help them address their type A personalities. After four years, the men who received treatment for their hostility, anger, and other type A factors had suffered fewer secondary heart attacks.

Another study, done by Dr. Dean Ornish—now famous for his heart disease rehabilitation program, which includes a low-fat diet, yoga, exercise, stress reduction, and social support—supports this belief. To help prove the authenticity of his approach, Ornish studied forty-one people with heart disease. Some received routine cardiac care; others got that same care as well as Ornish's complete treatment program: a low-fat diet, exercise, yoga, relaxation training, and stress-coping sessions. Those who received the additional training were able to reverse their heart disease: their coronary blockages actually shrank.

It's not clear that you can transform yourself from a hostile personality type into a calm one, but you can learn to manage these traits. Dr. Williams began studying hostility syndrome based on his own anger issues, and he's the first to admit that he must continue to work at staying calm.

Hostility may be a lot like an addiction. For instance, an alcoholic is never cured but is forever recovering. Recognizing that you need to change is a huge step in the right direction. You can change your cynical thoughts, lift your mood, calm your stress, and generally improve your life with a combined approach I teach in Chapters 7 through 9. It is worth trying. You will improve your overall health and likely extend your life by managing the hostile traits that most likely contribute to your diabetes.

Part II

The Program

6

Test Your Personality

Find the Optimal Mind-Body Program for You

THE chapters in Part II present two mind-body techniques designed to help you eliminate the mental barriers to blood sugar control. These are the same skills we teach that have been tested at Duke and other universities with great success. In Chapter 7, you will learn a highly effective way to relax called progressive muscle relaxation. In Chapter 8, you'll discover cognitive behavior therapy, which will help ease depression, hostility, and anxiety. Then in Chapter 9, you'll find out how to incorporate one or both techniques into a simple six-week program.

Must you learn both progressive muscle relaxation and cognitive behavior therapy? The answer to that question depends on your emotional, psychological state. To determine how best to proceed, you must first find out where you are now. That's what this chapter is about. The series of quizzes that you will take in this chapter will help you determine whether you are suffering from stress-induced rises in blood sugar, depression, or hostility syndrome:

- If you test low on every quiz in this chapter, you probably need to work on only the progressive muscle relaxation technique described in Chapter 7.
- If you test high for stress and either depression or hostility, then I recommend that you combine the techniques described in Chapters 7 and 8.

- If you test high for depression and not for hostility or stress, you may focus on just the technique in Chapter 8.

Your answers in the following quizzes will do more than help you see specifically which problems you most need to address. They will also help you to gauge your progress in learning these new skills. Take these quizzes now, and take them again in six weeks, after you've completed the step-by-step program outlined in Chapter 9. Compare the results to see how far you've come. These quizzes will also help you find out whether you need professional help or medication.

Before we get to the quizzes, let's first assess your readiness to tackle any life change.

THE STAGES OF CHANGE

The first question to ask yourself is, "Am I ready to tackle any program?" You may have already tried numerous strategies to improve your health and mental well-being. Some may have worked; others didn't. You may have stuck with some and not with others. Why do some approaches fail and others succeed? Your readiness for change may have more to do with your success than the specifics of your goal.

James O. Prochaska, Ph.D., director of the Cancer Prevention Research Consortium and professor of clinical and health psychology at the University of Rhode Island, has spent much of his career studying what helps people successfully make important health changes. Prochaska's father died of alcoholism and depression while Prochaska was in college studying to be a psychologist. His father had distrusted psychology to his dying day, and Prochaska wanted to understand why.

Wanting to make psychology more helpful to people like his dad, he explored why some patients seem to have great success and others do not and how some people are able to change negative behaviors and adopt positive ones and others cannot.

Prochaska searched for patterns among people who had already made behavior changes, particularly those who had successfully given up smoking. He learned that change is a process rather than a destination—a process that lasts many months, even years. During that process, someone might relapse or slip up numerous times, but as long as he sticks with the process, he eventually makes the new change a habit or leaves behind the old negative behavior.

In the late 1970s, Prochaska, along with Carlo DiClemente, Ph.D., now at the University of Maryland, came up with a model called the stages of change to help explain why some people seem to adopt new habits easily while others experience great difficulty. According to his theory, people trying to adopt new health habits go through the following six predictable stages:

1. PRECONTEMPLATION. If you are in this stage, you do not plan to make a significant change anytime during the next six months. You have not yet decided that a change is needed. You may actively look for reasons not to change. You may even be in denial, not believing the health consequences of diabetes, for example. Because you are reading this book, you probably have already moved beyond this stage.

2. CONTEMPLATION. In this stage, you intend to do something about your health and well-being within the next six months. You are aware of how your emotional habits are hurting your health. You realize that you need to do something but are not quite sure how to go about it or how long it will take you. You do not feel as if you need to do something about it tomorrow or today.

3. PREPARATION. In this stage you intend to do something within the next thirty days. You have already taken some steps to prepare for that change, such as reading this book. Once you get to the preparation stage, you have mentally committed yourself to doing something. You see the change as needed and positive, and you are ready to take steps to make it happen in your life.

4. ACTION. Once you get to this step, you are in the process of creating a change. The biggest mistake people make is not sticking with it long enough. To plant a new change in your life and be sure that it takes root, you must perform this action for at least six months. From day 1 to six months, you are at the highest risk for relapsing and returning to your old habits.

5. MAINTENANCE. Once you reach this stage, you have made a change more than 6 months ago. During this stage, you continue to work to solidify your new habits. You may slip up from time to time. For example, you may not practice your mini-relaxation sessions on certain days, or you may blow up at someone and allow yourself to slip back into an angry mood. These are not failures as long as you point yourself back in the right direction. The process of change can require months or even years of vigilance.

6. TERMINATION. You have safely adopted a new health habit or stopped a negative health habit and no longer need to worry about relapse. Though this stage is certainly the ideal, remember that many people spend their lives in the maintenance phase.

Seeing change as a process helps to soothe away the guilt of relapse. You see that the action and maintenance stages take time. During those stages, you may slip up from time to time. That's fine—it's part of the process. Just make sure you get yourself back on track.

WHAT STAGE ARE YOU IN?

To find out whether you are ready to tackle the program, answer the following questions:

1. Are you planning to change in the next six months?
2. Are you planning to change in the next thirty days?
3. Have you already made a change in the past twelve months?

To find out how you scored, consult the answer key on page 72.

If you are still in the precontemplation stage, you will have a difficult time tackling the program successfully. I suggest that you spend some time thinking about the pros and cons of tackling the program. Be honest. Include not only the pros and cons for you personally, but also how your change affects others you love. For example, remember that diabetes robs you of the energy you need to be a good parent or spouse. Hostility causes you to yell at your spouse and children. They have as much to gain by your getting help as you do. Reread Chapters 1 to 5 to remind yourself of the health challenges that you face if you don't tackle the program.

Once you have moved beyond the precontemplation stage, you are ready to take additional quizzes to determine your most important mind-body challenge: stress, depression, or hostility. The purpose of the following quizzes is not to give you a psychiatric diagnosis but to identify which areas of change you should focus on. Our research at Duke has shown that most people with diabetes, even those who do not consider themselves to be suffering from stress, can benefit from this program. Let's start by seeing how prone you are to stress.

Test Your Stress Response

Just about everyone can benefit from the stress management program described in Chapter 7. My research shows that stress management helps improve blood sugar even in people who wouldn't necessarily be characterized as highly stressed or abnormally anxious. To determine how much of a problem anxiety and stress are for you, I have compiled an informal test to help you make this assessment. Please answer the following questions as they pertain to the last seven days.

1. Do you feel anxious most of the time?
2. Do you feel easily rattled?
3. Do you find yourself worrying all the time?
4. Do you feel that your nerves are shot?
5. Do you feel that you handle things adequately?
6. Are you easily confused?
7. Do you worry a lot?
8. Are you insecure?
9. Are you often frightened?
10. Do you feel rested?
11. Do you feel tense all of the time?
12. Do you have disturbing thoughts?
13. Do you take your work problems home with you?
14. Are you unhappy?
15. Do you feel you can't unwind easily?

To find out how you did, turn to page 72 to learn if stress is a major problem for you.

Test Your Depression Level

Many people suffer from mild forms of depression that may go unnoticed by them or by others. Even health care providers can miss it. Depression is a serious condition that robs you of the joy of life and increases the risk of developing many diseases such as diabetes. It also increases the severity of such diseases. Severe forms of depression can lead to suicide.

Depression is a serious illness, and very specific psychological tests have been constructed to diagnose depression. The following questions are not meant to provide a diagnosis, but they can help you tell if you might be suffering from depression. With that information, you can start to address the problem.

To test whether you suffer from depression, answer the following questions as they pertain to the past seven days. Then turn to page 72 to learn if you suffer from depression and, if so, what you should do about it, including whether you should seek professional help.

1. Do you feel sad most of the time?
2. Do you often feel as if there's little to look forward to?
3. Do you see your life as being one failure after another?
4. Do you feel as if you no longer enjoy any activities these days?
5. Do you feel disgusted with yourself or hate yourself?
6. Do you feel that you have lost interest in sex?
7. Do you ever think of ending it all and just killing yourself?
8. Do you cry often?
9. Do you often feel irritated?
10. Do you feel as if there are very few people whom you enjoy being around?
11. Do you have trouble making decisions?
12. Do you feel as if there's nothing you feel like accomplishing?

13. Do you sleep poorly?
14. Do you feel fatigued most of the time?
15. Do you feel that you have lost your appetite?

Test Your Hostility Level

Although hostility is not a disease or disorder, specific psychological tests have been constructed to measure it. You can test your hostility level by answering the following questions.

1. When people tell you what to do, do you often feel as if they don't know what they are talking about?
2. When people tell you about a hardship they have encountered, do you often feel as if they are just trying to get attention?
3. When you argue with people, is it because they are always wrong?
4. Do you feel that most people would do anything to get ahead, including lying and stabbing others in the back?
5. Do you feel that the only time most people tell the truth is when they fear someone will know that they are lying?
6. Do you feel that most people are dishonest?
7. Do you feel that the only person you can count on is you?
8. Do you trust very few people?
9. Do you feel that most people use their friends for their personal gain?
10. Do you feel that few people like helping others?
11. Do you think that to survive in this world, you must live by the philosophy of "every man out for himself"?
12. Do you think that, if they knew they wouldn't get caught, most people would cheat on their spouses or have an affair with a married person?
13. Can you think of at least one person who is out to get you?
14. When someone compliments you, do you wonder what she or he wants you to do in return?
15. Do people treat you badly when you haven't done anything wrong?

To find out how you did, consult the "Scoring Key for Hostility" below.

Scoring Key for Stages of Change

If you answered: no to all questions, you are in the *precontemplation stage;* yes to #1, and no to #2 and #3, you are in the *contemplation stage;* yes to #1 and #2, and no to #3, you are in the *preparation stage;* yes to all questions, you are in the *action stage*.

Scoring Key for Stress

If you answered yes to five or more questions, stress is a problem in your life. You will benefit most by learning both progressive muscle relaxation and cognitive behavior therapy in tandem. If you answered yes to fewer than five questions, stress is not much of an issue for you, but you will probably still benefit from learning the technique in Chapter 7. If you answered yes to ten or more questions, stress is a major problem, and you should consider seeking help from a trained professional if the stress management techniques in this book do not work for you. See Chapter 13 for help on finding professional assistance.

Scoring Key for Depression

If you answered yes to five of the above questions, you're a good candidate for the cognitive behavior therapy technique in Chapter 8. If you answered yes to ten or more items, or any number of items including item 7, I suggest that you seek professional help, as a self-help program may not be sufficient to treat your depression. Depression is a serious illness, but it can be treated. For help on finding a trained professional, see Chapter 13.

Scoring Key for Hostility

If you answered yes to eight or more of these questions, you have a problem with hostility that can benefit from the cognitive behavior therapy technique in Chapter 8.

7

Progressive Muscle Relaxation

Six Steps to Stress Relief and Better Blood Sugar Control

I first experienced the benefits of progressive muscle relaxation during the 1970s as I was finishing my studies at McGill University. At the time, I wasn't studying it as a researcher. I was a patient.

I had developed a severe fear of flying after being on a flight from Montreal to New York during which the plane had trouble shortly after takeoff. I still vividly remember the flight attendant's announcing that something was wrong with the plane and the pilot had to make an emergency landing. She didn't provide many details, but her face was pale and pinched. I knew that something major must be wrong.

I don't remember feeling especially panicked at the time, and as it turned out, the landing proved uneventful. We didn't have to sit in a crouched position and didn't land on a highway or some strange location. The pilot simply went back to the Montreal airport, where the mechanics adjusted something and the plane took off again. The rest of the trip was uneventful. Within a few days, I had forgotten about the incident, or so I thought. Nine months later, I flew from Montreal to visit family in New York. On the return flight, I had a panic attack. As I sat in my seat, the incident that had happened months earlier flashed through my mind. My palms began to sweat, my heart raced, and my breathing became shallow and rapid. Although I had flown dozens of times before without any problem, I had become afraid to fly. When the plane finally touched down in Montreal, I knew I needed to address my anxiety.

During my training in clinical psychology, I had learned how to treat such simple fears or phobias. The technique is simple. Train the patient how to relax very deeply. Then ask the patient to imagine himself or herself in progressively more threatening situations. Eventually, the patient practices the relaxation skills in the real-life phobic situation. I began to practice the relaxation techniques myself, beginning each session by tensing and then relaxing my muscles, bringing myself to a state of deep calm. Then I imagined myself on an airplane. I would visualize a flight only to the point of feeling anxious, and then I would again focus on relaxing. After each session, I felt as if I had been drugged. I was amazed at the effect. After I could visualize an entire trip without feeling anxious, I decided it was time to fly and made it through the trip without a problem.

Several years later, I joined a colleague, Dr. Albert Forgione, and developed a workshop, in collaboration with Pan American Airlines, for people afraid to fly. Flying was no longer a problem for me. In fact, I went on to get my pilot's license and instrument rating.

Now, more than thirty years later, I know that relaxation techniques are important for many other reasons besides getting over simple phobias. These techniques can dramatically lower stress hormone levels for the long term, helping to prevent and treat numerous conditions from heart disease to headaches, circulatory problems to diabetes.

HOW RELAXATION HELPS

We've shown over and over again at Duke that practicing relaxation on a regular basis will improve blood sugar control. There are many ways to induce the relaxation response, and researchers have studied most of them, from meditation and deep breathing to prayer and drugs, all of which lower levels of stress hormones. Other relaxation methods have been used to help treat numerous diseases, including high blood pressure, cardiac arrhythmias, Raynaud's disease, and migraine headache, but I have found that progressive muscle relaxation is the best technique for most people. It is easiest to learn and the most convenient to incorporate into daily life.

All relaxation techniques work on the same basic principle: they trigger the relaxation response. Relaxation counters the body's fight-or-flight response, training you to turn it off. When you relax, you lower the levels of stress hormones in your blood, which results in decreased muscle tension, blood pressure, heart rate, and blood sugar. In short, your relaxation response is an antidote to your fight-or-flight response. Lowering levels of stress hormones will help keep the liver from overproducing sugar, allow the pancreas to release insulin in the right amounts, and thereby control your blood sugar.

In progressive muscle relaxation, you systematically tense and then relax the muscles in your body. Progressive muscle relaxation is the same technique that I taught Janice, the patient who was able to save her eyesight, and the preacher, who calmed blood sugar surges during his sermons, and that I learned to get over my fear of flying. It works for almost everyone. It's also possibly the most researched and effective of all the stress management techniques for diabetes as well as for other stress-related diseases. In a study many years ago, I compared progressive muscle relaxation to biofeedback and meditation for their effectiveness in treating high blood pressure. We trained patients in each technique for eight sessions. All the techniques led to lower blood pressure, but subjects had a much easier time learning and performing progressive muscle relaxation than the other techniques.

Until recently, I had used this technique only in hospital settings, teaching it to patients with a biofeedback machine and lots of one-on-one attention. While biofeedback is helpful for many patients, our research at Duke has shown that it is clearly not necessary for people to learn relaxation effectively.

Anyone can learn this technique without extensive one-on-one attention from a therapist or psychologist. During the mid-1990s at Duke, we studied 108 people with type 2 diabetes who underwent five group therapy sessions with or without stress management training. The sessions were simple and combined relaxation with some of the cognitive behavior therapy techniques provided in Chapter 8. The patients received an audiotape that contained the same instructions for relaxation as described on pages 87 to 96. They also received a booklet with instructions on how to use the tape to relax—the same instructions I provide shortly. The booklet explained how to use the technique and integrate it into their daily lives. We tried to provide as little instruction as we could, because we wanted to see if the method could be taught to people in a nonclinical setting. In other words, we wanted to see if people could learn mostly on their own.

As usual, for about six months, both groups benefited. This happens because people "get religion" when they enroll in a study. They attend to their diets and take their medications regularly, and everyone improves. That's why we followed people for a year. By six months, the groups began to diverge.

After one year, those who practiced progressive relaxation and followed the program had a 0.5 percent improvement in HbA_{1C}, a measure of long-term blood sugar control. Although that sounds like a very small reduction in blood sugar, this small degree of change is enough to reduce risk significantly for diabetes-related complications such as eye and kidney disease. Furthermore, nearly a third experienced much larger improvements of 1 percent or more. Most compelling was that the technique worked for everyone, including those who didn't initially test high on anxiety scales.

HOW TO RELAX

Learning to relax is simple. Most people don't need the help of a therapist or therapy group. They need only practice progressive muscle relaxation on a regular basis. I describe how to do other relaxation techniques in Chapter 12 so you can give them a try too. Even though you may find that you prefer another method, I suggest that you start with progressive muscle relaxation because it is the easiest to learn and the one that has been tested most often in diabetes. If you have the time and the interest, try them all eventually and see how they work for you. You want a method that works for you. It's that simple. Your goal is learning how to relax. Precisely how you take yourself from a stressed state to a relaxed state largely depends on your personality and lifestyle.

No matter what technique you use to bring yourself to a relaxed state, follow these pointers:

• KEEP YOUR MIND OPEN. Your attitude about relaxation is important. If you try it with an open mind, you will achieve better results. You must allow relaxation to unfold naturally. You can't force it. If you're type A, this may be hard. You may stress yourself by wondering, "Am I doing it right?" Sometimes people find the exercises are not working as well as they might like, so they try harder. This only makes matters worse. You relax by getting rid of pressures, not by adding to them. Relaxation is a process of letting go and learning to trust your body. Some people try to force control, which may increase anxiety. Take it easy, and do not try too hard. The more passive your attitude is, the more easily you will relax.

• EMPTY DISTRACTING THOUGHTS FROM YOUR MIND. You won't completely quiet your mind; your thoughts will drift from the relaxation exercise to something else from time to time, but don't focus on them. Allow them to pass through your mind like clouds.

• PRACTICE, PRACTICE, PRACTICE. This is key to your success. Relaxation is a learned process that takes time and effort. You'll start with 15 to 20 minutes twice a day. The more you practice, the more you will train your parasympathetic nervous system to relax, and the better able you'll be to relax automatically when you encounter a tense situation.

When you find yourself stuck in a long line at the supermarket, sitting in traffic, or not being able to reach someone on the phone, take a deep breath and practice relaxation. Concentrate on relaxation for 30 seconds and then return to normal life. These 30-second "mini-practices" will help you to be able to relax automatically whenever you need to. There's more about mini-practices on p. 85. Most people notice minor annoyances many times a day. By week 3 of the program, I'll ask you to try to complete twenty mini-practices a day. At the end of the day, record how many times you practiced. (I've provided you with a planner in Chapter 9 to do this record keeping). This will help make relaxation a regular habit.

• RELAX IN A QUIET SPACE. Get rid of all possible distractions before you attempt to relax. Turn off the television, radio, and other sources of noise. Turn off the telephone ringer, or take the phone off the hook. Turn off your pager or cell phone. Ask family members not to disturb you during relaxation. You might also enlist their help in handling any unforeseen distractions that may pop up, such as answering the door or quieting your barking dog.

• START FRESH. At least for the first week or two, relax during a time of day when you feel energetic. Too often people associate relaxation with fatigue. What your body feels as it drifts off to sleep (or attempts to drift off to sleep) and what you feel as you practice relaxing may seem similar at first, but there are some important differences. Relaxation is not the same thing as sleep.

When you are relaxed, your mind is active. You are able to think clearly and learn quickly. When you are fatigued, your mind is dull and inactive, and it is more difficult to take in new information. Practicing at a time of day when you feel energetic will allow you to master the relaxation technique more easily. It will also prevent the tendency to fall asleep. If you find that you do drift off to sleep when you practice your relaxation exercises, set an alarm clock to wake yourself.

• DO THE EXERCISES, NOT SOME OTHER ACTIVITY. Some people claim that they relax by watching television or by reading the newspaper, but blanking out in front of the TV or going to sleep at the end of a tiring day is not the same kind of relaxation you need to reduce stress and lower blood sugar. Practice progressive muscle relaxation regularly, and you will soon understand the difference between true relaxation and napping or television watching.

• COOL DOWN YOUR MIND. Tension creates a vicious cycle: the tenser you are, the harder it is to relax. If you begin by lowering the background levels of stress, you will find it easier to do the exercises. You will learn to relax and relax to learn. If you are especially tense, you may need to do more than settle down in a quiet space for a few minutes during the day before attempting your relaxation exercises. Some people find that a warm bath helps them calm down enough to try relaxation and concentrate on their exercises. You can try sitting quietly and listening to soft music. This will allow you to focus your mind on the exercise and prevent random thoughts from distracting your practice.

• SIT; DON'T LIE. Many people fall asleep during relaxation if they lie down. With some practice, you may be able to keep your focus and prevent yourself from falling asleep while lying on your back. In the beginning, however, practice your relaxation exercises while comfortably seated in a chair. Use a chair that supports your back. You don't need arm rests. You can rest your hands in your lap.

• GET COMFORTABLE. In the beginning, you'll be spending a half-hour on your relaxation exercises, so sit in a position that you find comfortable enough to maintain for 30 minutes without discomfort. Though you don't need special clothing to relax, wearing comfortable clothing, without shoes, will make it easier.

As you relax, your eyelids or limbs may feel heavy and you may breathe more slowly and deeply. Your hands and feet may get warmer, and you may notice your heart beating. (Body sounds are always present, but they are usually drowned out by our attention to outside events. With deep relaxation, even body sounds eventually recede from awareness.) Since you relax in gradual steps, you may not experience all of these sensations, but if you do feel them, do not be alarmed. You will never relax too deeply or too quickly. There is no danger at all in this exercise.

• GO SLOWLY. Do not hurry to get through your relaxation exercises. Nothing is more self-defeating than putting yourself under artificial time constraints.

Now that you know the basic rules of relaxation, let's move on to specifics about progressive muscle relaxation.

HOW PROGRESSIVE MUSCLE RELAXATION WORKS

At the turn of the century, Harvard physician Edmund Jacobson developed the first progressive muscle relaxation techniques. Jacobson believed that anxiety and other mental diseases are caused by tight, clenched muscles throughout the body, and so he developed a technique that involves tensing and then relaxing muscles systematically. Jacobson also noted that when patients were taught to relax their muscles, many of the physiological effects associated with stress and the fight-or-flight response decreased.

Muscle tension is often associated with the effects of stress, including increased heart rate, blood pressure, and stress hormone levels. Your body retains muscular control without your awareness. If this were not so, you would spend all of your time thinking about the changing state of your muscles. If you sat down to relax, you would find yourself focusing on the muscle tension in your abdomen and buttocks, without which you could not sit upright. If you tried to take a relaxing walk, your conscious mind would be so busy processing information on the forces applied to your muscles and on the required muscular reaction to deal with these forces that you would quickly become a nervous wreck.

Because your muscles adapt to tension, you lose the ability over time to notice tension. You notice it only when the tension is so high that it produces migraine headaches, neck or back pain, and other symptoms. Although adaptation lets us function more or less automatically in some situations, it is a mixed blessing. Over a prolonged period of stress or during shorter periods of severe stress, your body will adapt to the high levels of muscle tension. You continue to function, often unaware that you are in an abnormally high state of stress. Thus, the feedback signals that normally inform your nervous system to take it easy go unnoticed due to this adaptive process.

The reason for the inability to relax during such extreme tension is based on a well-known principle of perception. To understand this principle, stand in a brightly lit room and look at a white wall. Now strike a match. The room is unquestionably brighter because you just added a new source of light, but the total illumination in the room is so great, and the difference made by adding the light of the match so tiny, that you will notice no change in the illumination. If you lower the lights in the same room, you will see quite a different effect when you strike the match. This time, you will see the flickering match light up the walls. When the total illumination is low enough, you can easily see the change that the match causes.

It's the same way with relaxation and muscle tension. The greater the tension is in our muscles, the less we can sense any easing of that tension. Because muscles relax in gradual steps, we sometimes cannot notice the change at all if we are very tense. As a result, we are often least able to relax precisely at the times when we most need to.

Muscle movements and tension are controlled by the central nervous system, and although it may seem that we move our muscles automatically, their activity is obviously under voluntary control. Biofeedback studies have shown that people can be taught to manipulate their arteries, heart rate, and intestines, all of which are governed by the autonomic nervous system. When you relax your muscles, you calm the autonomic nervous system, which includes the levels of stress hormones and their effects on metabolism.

Because we are much more aware of the state of our muscles than we are of our levels of stress hormones, tuning in to muscle tension and reducing it is a sort of natural biofeedback. Few of us readily sense changes in our heart rates, but all of us can learn to feel changes in muscle tension. When you control your muscle tension, you reap the changes in your heart rate, blood pressure, and stress hormones as well.

When you practice progressive muscle relaxation, you will focus your attention on the way your muscles feel when they are tense and when they are relaxed. Tensing and then relaxing muscle groups will help you to gain this awareness. You will associate the word *relax* with this process, using it as a command or cue to relax your body. With practice and repetition, you will learn to keep your muscles relaxed on a regular basis.

Progressive muscle relaxation will teach you to release muscle tension, which will relax your entire body and mind. This will relieve tension and improve your blood sugar control and your overall health and well-being.

LEARNING PROGRESSIVE MUSCLE RELAXATION

You can learn progressive muscle relaxation within several weeks with the instructions in this book. All it takes is listening to the recorded instructions. You can create a tape by reading the scripts on pages 87 to 96 into a tape recorder or purchase the CD that we have used at Duke, available at www.richardsurwit.com. You'll eventually wean yourself off the tape or CD so that you can remind yourself silently how to relax, almost instantly.

On the scripts and the CD, I've combined progressive muscle relaxation with a technique called guided imagery, a complementary relaxation technique that has been used to treat many ailments, including high blood pressure, irregular heartbeat, anxiety, and sexual problems. The relaxation exercises will help fully relax your body, but you can enter a state of even deeper relaxation by combining them with mental imagery. Related to self-hypnosis, imagery relies on images rather than words and has been used in all sorts of ways, from an asthma patient's imagining wide-open lung passages to cancer patients' seeing their immune systems attack their tumors. For your own relaxation exercise, the script asks you to imagine a leaf falling slowly to the ground.

Imagery is more than just seeing images in your mind's eye. It involves all of your senses. You will try to hear, feel, taste, and smell what you are imagining. The more vividly you imagine something, the more real it seems to the brain. In fact, you can also use imagery to practice and improve golf swings, tennis serves, pitching and batting, and other athletic activities.

Visual, auditory, and tactile images stem from the brain's cerebral cortex. Position emission tomography (PET) scans show that imagining a scene produces the same changes in the brain as actually seeing or experiencing it. Depending on the image, the brain signals different parts of the body to calm down or fight or flee. This is why you can watch a movie of a roller-coaster ride and feel the same drop in the pit of your stomach as if you were really on the roller coaster. The message travels from your cerebral cortex to your hypothalamus to your endocrine glands.

Here are some tips for getting started on your progressive muscle relaxation program:

• Start each session by mentally assessing your tension level and or pain intensity. How are you feeling at this moment? Rate your tension level on a scale from 1 to 10, with 1 feeling peaceful and 10 feeling panic. Record these values in your daily planner in Chapter 9. After your session, again rate your tension level on a 1 to 10 scale. Such measures will help you to realize the benefits of relaxation as you practice and reach greater degrees of relaxation.

• Practice relaxation on a regular basis at scheduled times. Your planner in Chapter 9 will help keep you on track. At first, your sessions will last 15 to 20 minutes, twice a day. As you advance through the program, you'll be able to use the technique to relax your body automatically within seconds.

• During week 3, begin to use these techniques when you feel stress and tension. Once you notice sweaty palms, a headache, achy muscles, a racing heart, or panicked thoughts, do a 30-second mini-relaxation session.

• In your daily planner in Chapter 9, keep a record of your frequency of practice. It does not matter how you choose to remind yourself to relax. What is important is that you practice frequently. Little by little, you can develop the habit of keeping yourself relaxed throughout the day.

Is It Working?

The most reliable way to see if you are relaxing properly is to take your pulse rate before and after each session. You can find your pulse most easily at your wrist or on your neck, just below the point where your jaw meets your neck. Count the number of heartbeats over 15 seconds (you'll need a second hand) and then multiply by 4. If you are relaxing properly (and if you don't have a pacemaker or are not on cardiac-blocking drugs), your pulse will drop by about 10 beats per minute, with bigger drops as you become more adept at relaxation.

Testing whether relaxation is lowering your blood sugar over the short term is a bit trickier. Your blood sugar will change with your weight, how much activity you are engaging in, and what you have just eaten, and if any of these things are fluctuating, they may mask the effects of relaxation. If you adhere to the program and don't put on weight, however, you should see your fasting blood sugar, as well as your blood sugar after meals, start to come down after about six weeks. These changes should be especially noticeable right after you have practiced relaxing. After 12 weeks you should see a change in your HbA_{1C}.

YOUR PROGRESSIVE MUSCLE RELAXATION TIMELINE

During weeks 1 through 3, you will practice progressive muscle relaxation in formal 30-minute sessions. After that, you will work on monitoring your stress and tension levels and then use progressive muscle relaxation mini-practice sessions to bring yourself to a calm state. Follow these practice instructions for 6 weeks and beyond:

Week 1. Listen to script 1 twice a day at times that fit your schedule. Relax, and maintain a passive attitude while letting your body follow the instructions you are giving it. Remember to record your tension levels before and after each relaxation session in your daily planner.

Week 2. Continue listening to script 1 once a day. In addition, begin practicing with script 2, preferably later in the day. This second script does not involve tensing and releasing your muscles. Instead, you will go through all of the muscle groups and try to relax them without tensing them first. Practicing script 2 will help you to learn to relax any time and prepare you for the exercises in week 3.

Week 3. Stop listening to script 1 and listen instead to script 2 once a day. Begin your mini-practices, 30 to 60 seconds at a time (see the section that follows, "Mini-Practices 101") when you notice that you're becoming tense.

Weeks 4, 5, 6, and Beyond. Continue your mini-practices, aiming for twenty 30- to 60-second sessions a day. You may continue formal 20-minute relaxation sessions if you choose, but they are not required.

MINI-PRACTICES 101

Mini-practices are just that: very brief periods—30 seconds—where you focus on your muscle tension and try to relax. During a mini-practice, you'll quickly perform a mental scan of the major muscle groups that you've learned to attend to in progressive muscle relaxation. By the time you have practiced for two weeks, you will be able to go from head to toe quite quickly. If you notice any tension in any of the muscle groups, say the word *relax* to yourself, and let that tension go.

Mini-practices are the key to making progressive relaxation work for you. Relaxing twice a day is beneficial, but it will not affect your blood sugar over the course of a whole day. For progressive relaxation to work to keep your blood sugar down, you must keep your levels of stress hormones down throughout the day.

The way to incorporate mini-practices into your daily routine is to create a simple cue to remind yourself to do a mini-practice. At Duke, we tell patients to buy a box of little stickers that they can place around their environment that will remind them to do a mini-practice. These stickers can be little stars, dots, or sticky notes. Anything small with a self-adhesive backing will do. You can usually find a wide variety of these items in a drugstore or any office supply store. Place the stickers where you will see them: on your computer monitor, your TV screen, your refrigerator, the dashboard of your car, your bathroom mirror, or any other visible place. They can be placed discreetly so that only you notice them. The telephone is a good place to put one, but use it to remind yourself to relax before you make a call, not while you try to answer a ringing phone!

Each time you find yourself becoming tense, pay attention to where these feelings of stress or tension are in your body. Each time you encounter an annoying situation, stop yourself, take a long breath, and say the word *relax* to yourself. Slowly exhale, and while you are doing so, concentrate on the sensations of relaxation within your body. No matter what you are doing, stop for about 30 seconds to allow yourself to relax and focus on the sensations of increasing relaxation.

Allow your jaw to relax, and allow sensations of heaviness to flow from your shoulders down through your body. Make sure that you are breathing from the abdomen.This will help you to stay relaxed.

After 30 seconds have passed, return to whatever activity you were engaged in regardless of how well you have succeeded in achieving relaxation. Never extend your mini-practice session beyond 1 minute. If you do not feel relaxed, nevertheless continue with what you were doing and stop yourself the next time an annoying situation reminds you to practice. You will find that as you practice these mini-sessions, you will become better and better at producing sensations of relaxation in a short period of time.

Learning to produce relaxation quickly is similar to learning to shoot at a target or hit a baseball. Frequent practice is key. You will find that you will be able to feel increases in the relaxation response more reliably each time you practice.

Try to get up to thirty mini-practices a day. If you can do that, you will be spending only 15 minutes a day keeping yourself relaxed.

Now, it's time to relax.

Progressive Muscle Relaxation Scripts

Read the two scripts that follow into a tape or digital recorder. Read them slowly, pausing for 10 seconds between instructions. Don't read the word *pause* into the tape recorder. Rather, as you are reading the script, stop, say nothing, and wait for that specified amount of time. Many people find the sound of their own recorded voice annoying, usually because they are not used to hearing it. If the sound of your voice bothers you, you can ask a friend or relative to record the script for you, or you can simply order the relaxation CD. You can purchase the CD we use at Duke at www.richardsurwit.com

Script 1

Let your eyes drift shut, and settle down as best you can. For the next few moments, begin to adopt an attitude that nothing is of much importance other than concentrating on this exercise and relaxing.

PAUSE FOR 10 SECONDS

Begin by directing your attention to your feet.

PAUSE FOR 10 SECONDS

Slowly begin to bend both feet upward at the ankles, bringing the toes toward the knees. Build the tension slowly so that you can study it as it builds. Build the tension slowly under your control up to a point equally in both feet without hurting them.

PAUSE FOR 10 SECONDS

Now think the word *relax,* and slowly let the tension go. Study the relaxation as it goes into those muscles under your control, pleasantly deeper and deeper. Allow your feet to achieve their most comfortable position, allowing the relaxed muscles to find that position without your stretching them in the opposite direction.

PAUSE FOR 10 SECONDS

Focus your attention on the muscles of the thighs.

PAUSE FOR 10 SECONDS

Tense these muscles without lifting your legs so that your feet do not leave the floor. Concentrate on the building tension in your thighs. Build the tension, and study it.

PAUSE FOR 10 SECONDS

Think the word *relax*. Slowly let the tension go. Study the relaxation folding into your legs under your control. Let the relaxation flow deeper and deeper as your legs continue to relax.

PAUSE FOR 10 SECONDS

Focus your attention on your buttocks.

PAUSE FOR 10 SECONDS

Begin to tense them by pinching them together and folding them upward and inward, rolling your legs outward as you build the tension under your control. Feel yourself being lifted up by the increasing tension. Build the tension, and hold it.

PAUSE FOR 10 SECONDS

Think the word *relax,* and let the tension go. Feel the relaxation coming into those muscles under your control as if you were sinking into a soft cushion, pleasantly deeper and deeper. Let the chair support your weight. Let yourself relax completely.

PAUSE FOR 10 SECONDS

Try to follow the flow of relaxation a little deeper.

PAUSE FOR 10 SECONDS

Focus your attention on your abdomen.

PAUSE FOR 10 SECONDS

Begin to tense this sheet of muscle by slowly pulling the navel in toward the backbone. Continue to breathe more and more with the upper part of the chest building the tension under your control. Continue breathing with your chest and notice that you can continue to breathe regardless of where the tension is in your body. Hold the tension.

PAUSE FOR 10 SECONDS

Think the word *relax,* letting the abdomen sag, relaxing more and more under your control. It doesn't matter what you look like when you relax. What is important is that you are relaxing deeper and deeper.

PAUSE FOR 10 SECONDS

Notice that your breathing moves downward as this muscle relaxes. Abdominal breathing is relaxed breathing, slowly in and out, relaxing.

PAUSE FOR 10 SECONDS

Direct your attention to your hands.

PAUSE FOR 10 SECONDS

Begin to build the tension in both hands equally by pulling the fingertips and hands backward, bending both hands at the wrists back toward the elbow. Build the tension under your control in the back of the hand and the forearms. Hold that tension and study it.

PAUSE FOR 10 SECONDS

Think the word *relax*. Slowly let the tension go, and study the relaxation as it flows deeper and deeper under your control. You are relaxing your hands and arms deeper and deeper. Allow this sensation of relaxation to flow to the rest of the muscles in your body. Let the chair support your weight as you relax more and more deeply.

PAUSE FOR 10 SECONDS

Concentrate on the muscles in the back of your neck and shoulders.

PAUSE FOR 10 SECONDS

Begin by slowly raising your shoulders upward, letting your arms roll outward. At the same time, begin to tilt your head slowly backward, building the tension in the back and right between the shoulders. Do not force this exercise. Allow your mouth to open and breathe. Hold the tension.

PAUSE FOR 10 SECONDS

Think the word *relax,* and let the tension go. Feel the relaxation flow outward along the shoulders as they sag. Allow your head to tilt forward. Feel the relaxation up the back of your neck, spreading out over your back, spreading deeper and deeper. Your shoulders are dropping more and more. Your head is tilting more and more, relaxing. As your head comes forward, let it rest in whatever position is most comfortable.

PAUSE FOR 10 SECONDS

Bend your head forward, holding your chin toward your chest.

PAUSE FOR 10 SECONDS

Build the tension in the back of the neck, and hold it there. Study it.

PAUSE FOR 10 SECONDS

Think the word *relax,* and let the tension go, allowing your head to turn to a comfortable position.

PAUSE FOR 10 SECONDS

Tense your neck by bending your head to the right side, bending your right ear toward your right shoulder. Build the tension, but don't force it. Hold the tension like that and study it.

PAUSE FOR 10 SECONDS

Say the word *relax* to yourself, and let the tension go. Allow your head to return to a comfortably relaxed position.

PAUSE FOR 10 SECONDS

Bend your neck to the other side, moving your left ear toward your left shoulder. Again, build the tension and gently hold it there. Study the tension.

PAUSE FOR 10 SECONDS

Say the word *relax* to yourself, and let the tension go. Allow your head to come to rest in its most relaxed position.

PAUSE FOR 10 SECONDS

Focus your attention on your forehead.

PAUSE FOR 10 SECONDS

With your eyes still closed, begin to raise your eyebrows, wrinkling your forehead. You are building the tension in that part of your body under your control. Slowly build it up, and hold it there. Study the tension.

PAUSE FOR 10 SECONDS

Think the word *relax,* and slowly let the relaxation flow smoothly over the top of your head and down over the upper part of your face, making your face smoother and smoother while you relax.

PAUSE FOR 10 SECONDS

Now tense the muscles of your eyelids and the muscles around your eyes. Slowly and gently, shut your eyes tighter and tighter, though without excessive force, building the tension more and more. Then hold it there. Study the tension under your control.

PAUSE FOR 10 SECONDS

Think the word *relax,* letting the tension go. Relax, and feel the relaxation going deeper and deeper, as if it is dissolving the tension around the eyes.

PAUSE FOR 10 SECONDS

Begin to draw the corners of your mouth deeper and deeper into your cheeks, building the tension into a tight smile. Slowly build the tension and hold it. Study the tension.

PAUSE FOR 10 SECONDS

Think the word *relax,* studying the relaxation as it flows into the cheeks under your control. As it flows, allow your lips to part slowly and your jaw to sag, relaxing deeper and deeper with your tongue resting and your face expressionless. Continue relaxing for a moment or two, and enjoy the pleasant feeling in your body, which you have allowed to occur under your own control.

PAUSE FOR 10 SECONDS

Without force, begin a slow deepening of the breath all the way into a comfortable depth, all the way in comfortably and smooth.

PAUSE FOR 10 SECONDS

Think the word *relax,* and let the air flow out like the air out of a balloon. Let the air, not the muscles, do the work. Feel the pleasant, easy relaxing in your chest, relaxing deeper and deeper. Then let your body breathe at its own pace.

PAUSE FOR 10 SECONDS

While enjoying the relaxation, imagine the following scene.

PAUSE FOR 10 SECONDS

You are sitting outside in a comfortable lounge chair.

PAUSE FOR 10 SECONDS

You can feel the sun on your body. Your arms and legs are warm and heavy.

PAUSE FOR 10 SECONDS

Your whole body is comfortable and relaxed.

PAUSE FOR 10 SECONDS

In front of you is a tall, strong tree, with broad green leaves.

Notice that one leaf at the very top of the tree has become detached, and watch it as it drifts from side to side, drifting and settling effortlessly—so softly, so gently, that when it finally comes to rest, it will hardly bend a single blade of grass.

PAUSE FOR 10 SECONDS

Picture the leaf drifting and floating from side to side.

PAUSE FOR 10 SECONDS

Allow the leaf to come to rest now.

PAUSE FOR 10 SECONDS

Picture it quietly resting there.

PAUSE FOR 10 SECONDS

Its gentle weight is supported by the grass without the slightest strain, an effortless balance just as your body is supported by the chair.

PAUSE FOR 10 SECONDS

Enjoy the deep calm you have provided yourself.

PAUSE FOR 10 SECONDS

Each time you do this exercise, you become more and more familiar with the pattern of relaxation in your body.

PAUSE FOR 10 SECONDS

Your concentration becomes stronger, concentrating on the pattern of the elements of the exercise that allow the pattern of relaxation to emerge more and more.

PAUSE FOR 10 SECONDS

When you feel ready, begin to think of opening your eyes.

PAUSE FOR 10 SECONDS

From time to time, the feeling of wanting to stretch will come into your muscles.

Allow that feeling to occur.

PAUSE FOR 10 SECONDS

Notice how freely the breath moves into your lungs.

PAUSE FOR 10 SECONDS

Soon your eyelids begin to flutter.

PAUSE FOR 10 SECONDS

Allow them to, getting lighter and lighter, as if they want to open on their own.

PAUSE FOR 10 SECONDS

Any weight that was there dissolves.

PAUSE FOR 10 SECONDS

When they open, your eyes will be crystal clear and your senses crisp.

PAUSE FOR 10 SECONDS

When your eyes begin to open, notice that your body can be at ease and your mind active.

PAUSE FOR 10 SECONDS

Enjoy the benefits of relaxation that you have provided yourself. You can marshal your body for the tasks at hand at any time, but for a moment or two, enjoy the calm that you have produced under your control.

Script 2

Let your eyes drift shut, and settle down as best you can. For the next few moments, begin to adopt an attitude that nothing is of much importance other than concentrating on this exercise and relaxing.

PAUSE FOR 10 SECONDS

Begin by turning your attention to your feet.

PAUSE FOR 10 SECONDS

Do not tense your feet. Simply study their level of tension.

PAUSE FOR 10 SECONDS

Say the word *relax* to yourself, and slowly let any existing tension go. Study the relaxation as it comes into both calves under your control, pleasantly deeper and deeper. Simply allow your feet to relax.

PAUSE FOR 10 SECONDS

Focus your attention on the muscles of the thighs. Assess the amount of tension present in this part of your body. Study the tension without making any movement.

PAUSE FOR 10 SECONDS

Think the word *relax,* and let the tension go, studying the sensation as it flows into your legs under your control, deeper and deeper.

PAUSE FOR 10 SECONDS

As your legs continue to relax, focus your attention on your buttocks, and assess the amount of tension present in these large muscles.

PAUSE FOR 10 SECONDS

Say the word *relax* to yourself, and let the tension go. Feel the relaxation come into these muscles under your control, as if you were sinking into a soft cushion, pleasantly deeper and deeper. Let the chair support your weight, and try to follow the flow of relaxation just a little deeper.

PAUSE FOR 10 SECONDS

Focus your attention on your abdomen. Study the level of tension present in this muscle.

PAUSE FOR 10 SECONDS

Think the word *relax,* and allow the tension to disappear. Let your abdomen sag, relaxing more and more under your control. It doesn't matter what you look like when you relax. What is important is that you are relaxing deeper and deeper. Notice that your breathing moves downward as your relaxation deepens. Abdominal breathing is relaxed breathing.

PAUSE FOR 10 SECONDS

Direct your attention to your hands. Notice if any tension is present in the muscles of the hands and forearms.

PAUSE FOR 10 SECONDS

Think the word *relax,* and slowly let the tension go, allowing the relaxation to flow deeper and deeper from your hands into your arms and then into the rest of the muscles in your body.

PAUSE FOR 10 SECONDS

Concentrate on the muscles in the back of your neck and shoulders. Concentrate on any tension that might be present in these muscles.

PAUSE FOR 10 SECONDS

Study the tension, and then let these muscles relax under your control. Let your shoulders sag and come forward. Your shoulders are drooping more and more and your head is tilting more and more. As your head comes forward, let it rest in whatever position is most comfortable.

PAUSE FOR 10 SECONDS

Focus your attention on your forehead. Notice if any tension is present in this area; if there is, let it go under your control.

PAUSE FOR 10 SECONDS

As you relax, imagine your forehead becoming smoother and smoother, smoothing over the top of your head and down over the upper part of your face. Allow the relaxation to spread from the forehead into the muscles of the eyes and from the eyes into the muscles around the mouth. As your mouth relaxes, study the relaxation as it moves into your cheeks under your control. Allow your lips to part slowly, your jaw to sag, and your face to become expressionless as you relax deeper and deeper.

PAUSE FOR 10 SECONDS

Continue relaxing for a moment or two, and enjoy the feelings in your body that you have allowed to occur under your control.

PAUSE FOR 10 SECONDS

While enjoying the relaxation, imagine the following scene: You are sitting outside in a comfortable lounge chair.

PAUSE FOR 10 SECONDS

You can feel the sun on your body. Your arms and legs are warm and heavy. Your entire body is warm and relaxed.

PAUSE FOR 10 SECONDS

In front of you is a tall, strong tree covered with broad green leaves.

PAUSE FOR 10 SECONDS

Notice that one leaf at the very top of the tree has become detached, and watch it as it drifts from side to side, drifting and settling effortlessly, so softly, so gently, that when it finally comes to rest, it will hardly bend a single blade of grass.

PAUSE FOR 10 SECONDS

Picture the leaf drifting and floating from side to side.

PAUSE FOR 10 SECONDS

Allow the leaf to come to rest now.

PAUSE FOR 10 SECONDS

Picture it quietly resting there, its gentle weight supported by the grass without the slightest strain, an effortless balance just as your body is supported by the chair.

PAUSE FOR 10 SECONDS

Enjoy the deep calm you are providing yourself. Each time you do this exercise, you become more and more familiar with the pattern of relaxation in your body. Your concentration becomes stronger, concentrating on the elements of the exercise that allow the pattern of relaxation to emerge more and more.

PAUSE FOR 10 SECONDS

When you feel ready, begin to think of opening your eyes.

PAUSE FOR 10 SECONDS

From time to time, the feeling of wanting to stretch will come into your muscles. Allow that feeling to occur.

PAUSE FOR 10 SECONDS

Notice how freely the breath moves in your lungs.

PAUSE FOR 10 SECONDS

Soon your eyelids begin to flutter. Allow them to, becoming lighter and lighter as if they were about to open on their own. Any weight that was there dissolves. When they open, your eyes will be crystal clear and your senses crisp.

PAUSE FOR 10 SECONDS

As your eyes begin to open, notice that your body can be at ease and your mind active.

PAUSE FOR 10 SECONDS

Enjoy the benefits of relaxation you have provided yourself. You can marshal your body for the tasks at hand any time, but for a moment or two, enjoy the calm that you have produced under your control.

Source: Adapted from *Fear: Learning to Cope* (New York: Van Nostrand Reinhold, 1978), by Albert G. Forgione and Richard S. Surwit with Daniel G. Page. Copyright ©1978 by Albert G. Forgione, Richard S. Surwit, and Daniel G. Page.

8
Cognitive Behavior Therapy

Six Steps That Will Help You Relieve Anxiety,
Improve Your Mood, and Ease Hostility

STRESS is heightened by how we react mentally, as well as physically, to what happens to us. If you scored high on any of the quizzes in Chapter 6—anxiety, depression, or hostility—you may benefit from cognitive behavior therapy to help you achieve optimal blood sugar control. Research on cognitive behavior therapy clearly shows that this technique benefits patients with diabetes.

Versions of this type of therapy have been used by psychotherapists and counselors for many years. The earliest form of this therapy was developed by the well-known psychologist Albert Ellis in the 1950s and called rational emotive therapy. It focused on helping patients change irrational beliefs that motivated neurotic behavior. In the late 1960s, Canadian psychologist Donald Michenbaum established self-instructional training, which focused on how thoughts lead to specific behaviors, such as aggression. Finally, in the 1970s the psychiatrist Aaron Beck combined these techniques into what is now called cognitive behavior therapy and used it to treat depression.

Cognitive behavior therapy can dramatically improve your mood and overall outlook on life. In numerous studies, it has been found to be as effective as medication in treating depression. It's also the therapy of choice for people who have a problem with hostility. Most important, you don't necessarily need one-on-one sessions with a therapist to use it. Once you understand the basic technique, you can serve as your own therapist and find solutions to your problems.

Cognitive behavior therapy uses the difference between pessimists and optimists to show thought patterns and change them. Pessimists always see a partially filled glass as half empty, whereas optimists see it as half full. Cognitive behavior therapy teaches how to examine negative or irrational automatic thoughts and beliefs and replace them with positive, rational ones. Although negative thoughts and beliefs are often irrational, they are so ingrained and habitual that most of us don't even realize that we have them. For instance, in the parable of Chicken Little, the chick gets hit on the head with an acorn and immediately panics and believes the sky is falling. Chicken Little is a pessimist. Once you uncover your own pessimistic thoughts and beliefs, you test them to see for yourself how flawed they are. Then you will learn how to replace them with more accurate, positive views of yourself, other people, and the rest of the world.

Research shows that you can change your thoughts and beliefs, transforming yourself from a pessimistic person to an optimistic one. You can learn to lift yourself out of mild to moderate depression and soothe away anger. By doing this, you will also better control your blood sugar by preventing the fight-or-flight response from kicking in prematurely or unnecessarily. When you practice cognitive behavior therapy often enough, you'll eventually find that you will stay relaxed all the time because you've developed a healthy state of mind.

That's the cognitive part of the therapy. To improve your outlook on life, however, you also must change your behavior too. How you interact with others greatly influences how others treat you, which influences how you see them. Your thoughts, moods, and actions all affect each other.

To change your behavior, you'll learn to work with your social network and find out how friends, family, coworkers, and even your family doctor can help you remove pressure from your life and lower your overall stress level. You'll learn how speak up for your needs without feeling guilty and without angering others. You'll find solutions to problems, manage your time more effectively, and infuse your life with more meaning and balance.

To help you learn the technique, Chapter 9 includes daily reflective questions, tips, and reminders to help you stay on track. Each day, as you work through that chapter, you'll receive the tools you need to examine the automatic thoughts and behaviors that may be contributing to stress, anxiety, anger, or depression.

Before we get to the nuts and bolts of cognitive behavior therapy, however, let's first take a look at its track record for helping people improve their lives.

THE RESEARCH

Many people and even many physicians think of medication as the first therapy for depression, anxiety, and hostility. You'll learn more about the pros and cons of certain medications in Chapter 11. For now, however, let me assure you that drugs are not the only answer. For some people, they also may not be the best answer.

As you'll learn in Chapter 11, many mood-altering medications have side effects. Because each chemical in your brain performs numerous functions, altering any one brain chemical will alter more than just one part of your body. Although some people certainly benefit from medication (and you'll learn whether you are one of them in Chapter 11), many others simply need to learn how to change their perception of the world and their life.

Dozens of studies demonstrate the effectiveness of cognitive behavior therapy for depression, but its application to diabetes is more recent. One of the best studies on the benefits of cognitive behavior therapy for people with diabetes was done by noted depression and diabetes researcher Patrick Lustman, of Washington University in St. Louis, Missouri. Lustman and his colleagues studied fifty-one patients with type 2 diabetes who also had been diagnosed with major depression. About half of the patients took part in ten weeks of cognitive behavior therapy, and the other half did not. Not surprisingly, those in the cognitive behavior therapy group were more likely to experience a remission in their depression. Those who received the therapy had an 85 percent remission rate; those who did not had only a 27 percent remission rate. In addition, those who received cognitive behavior therapy also improved their blood sugar levels within six months of receiving the treatment.

A research paper published in *Diabetic Medicine* in 2002 reviewing existing studies dealing with psychological problems that affect people with diabetes—including depression, eating disorders, anxiety, stress, and interpersonal conflicts—found that cognitive behavior therapy consistently helped lift depression and improve blood sugar in people with type 2 diabetes.

HOW COGNITIVE BEHAVIOR THERAPY WORKS

How you see the world and view your problems makes a difference in how you respond and cope. For instance, if you see the world and the people in it as basically benign and good, you will generally see problems as temporary setbacks that you can easily solve. If you see the world as a dog-eat-dog competitive place and every person as selfish or out to get you, you will feel a lot more stress, anger, and depression. Cognitive behavior therapy will help you recognize your thought patterns and how they lead to moods or feelings, which lead to actions and behaviors. It shows you how changing your thoughts can change your mood and actions. Although moods may sometimes feel as if they arise all by themselves, they are usually connected to our thoughts, even if we don't quite notice the thoughts that lead to the moods.

How you interpret information will affect how you feel about life unfolding in front of you. For example, let's say your doctor is running behind schedule (as usual). You think, "No matter what, he makes me wait. Doesn't he think my time is as important as his?" You drum your fingers on the edge of your chair, sigh loud enough for the receptionist to hear, and frown at her. She senses your irritation and does her best to ignore you. You sigh some more. You get up and pace. You give the receptionist periodic dirty looks. She responds by leaving. "See, she doesn't even care that I have to wait," you think, and storm out of the office, skipping your appointment.

Let's take a look at it from a different angle. You notice that your doctor is running late, but instead you turn around your thoughts and say to yourself, "Okay, I've got some extra time. What can I do with it?" You look around the waiting room and see some medical literature on a table. You pick it up and read. You find out that a new drug has been approved to treat diabetes. You decide to ask your doctor about it.

The difference between the two situations lies in the thoughts that automatically pop up. Sometimes, of course, our thoughts are completely justified. Other times, they are exaggerated, distorted, and only half true. Once your thoughts start, they tend to travel in a particular pattern. If you are hostile, your pattern will include thoughts about the ways others have hurt or persecuted you. If you are depressed, your thoughts will focus on the hopeless nature of the world or on your personal faults and failures.

Let's take a look at how the technique might help someone with a hostile personality type. As you learned in Chapter 5, the first part of the hostility equation is cynicism. When you feel that someone has taken advantage of you, cynical thoughts pop up that fuel your anger, mobilizing the fight-or-flight response. Cynical thoughts about yourself, others, and the rest of the world make you prone to feeling anger. For example, your thoughts tell you that "all checkout cashiers are morons." As you stand in line at the checkout and the cashier has trouble ringing up an item, cynical thoughts start running through your mind. "Why don't these stores hire smarter people? Why don't they train them? Are they trying to ruin my day?" Your thoughts and anger show on your face and in your body language. The checkout person reads your body language and feels vulnerable and nervous, which makes him fumble some more, which makes you angrier.

You can see how the thoughts lead to the anger, which leads to behavior, which leads to others mistreating you, which leads to negative thoughts. Do you feel that your anger is always justified? Why do you get angry when standing in line at the grocery store and someone else does not? Perhaps you know someone who would get ticked off by something that wouldn't bother you at all.

What makes us angry often relates back to events that occurred earlier in our lives and our beliefs and thoughts about them. For many people, anger is a protective adaptation. Some people respond to abuse with rage, others with depression. The difference in response lies in the thoughts in your head.

To see this clearly, think back over your day or week to a time when you felt really angry. What was the situation? What thoughts ran through your mind as it was happening? Usually when we feel angry, the root of the anger is that we feel hurt or taken advantage of. Whether you get angry depends on how you interpret the information. You will anger quickly if you think the person meant to hurt you. If you think it was an accident, however, you may not be so quick to anger. You will most likely feel angry with people to whom you feel closest because you have a set of expectations about them. You may expect your husband *always* to listen to your problems or your kids *always* to do what they are told. You may expect your coworkers to get projects done on time. You may expect friends to understand your health problems and how they affect your life. When people don't live up to such expectations, you feel angry.

Depression also results from flawed thought processes. Aaron Beck showed in the 1960s that depression was caused at least in part by thought patterns that worked to strengthen and maintain a depressed mood. If you're depressed, you tend to think negative thoughts about yourself, other people, the world, and the future. Self-critical thoughts, such as, "I always screw things up" or "I'm undependable," contribute to low self-esteem and low self-confidence. This self-image affects how you deal with others and how they deal with you. Negative thoughts about the world may result in your thinking that others are thinking negative things about you when they really are not. You perceive others as mean and critical because you discount and ignore when they are positive and nurturing, which creates a vicious cycle. Your negative thoughts put you in a bad mood. Because of your negativity, others avoid you. Your lack of friends makes you think even more negatively.

Common thoughts that often run through the minds of people who are depressed include:

- I'm no good.
- Nobody loves me.
- Nobody understands me.
- I'm worthless.
- I can't get anything right.
- People can't depend on me.
- I let people down.
- Things will always be this way.
- I screwed up again.
- I can't change.
- I can't do anything about this.

Cognitive behavior therapy will help you to examine such thoughts and learn how to think more realistically. It may also help you better handle stress, particularly if you feel very anxious in certain situations, such as awaiting test results or helping your children with their homework. Though you may call it stress, anxiety often truly results from fear. Anxiety may result from a past traumatic event, parental conditioning, and life events and experiences. Often when you feel anxious, thoughts that accompany the anxiety magnify what you are feeling. Your thoughts tell you that you are in danger or that you are vulnerable. Anxious thoughts usually project you into the future; you worry about what may happen rather than what currently is happening. You're filled with "what ifs." Examining and replacing these anxious thoughts when necessary will help you to develop a better sense of safety in the present.

If mood or psychological problems are interfering with your blood sugar control, cognitive behavior therapy can help. It's a four-part process:

1. NOTICING YOUR MOODS. You will learn to go beyond "I'm in a good [or bad] mood," and pinpoint your moods with specific descriptions such as *angry, disappointed, frustrated,* and *anxious.* Once you understand your moods and notice when they start and stop, you will be able to pinpoint the thoughts that trigger them.

2. EXAMINING YOUR THOUGHTS. Once you understand your moods, you will work to uncover the thoughts that lead to them. Much of our thinking is so automatic that you may need to work even to notice your thoughts, but once you hear them, you'll clearly see how they affect your moods. Then you'll learn ways to examine them for accuracy, and, if needed, replace them with more realistic thoughts that will help you to boost your mood.

Of course, you can't just wipe away all negative thoughts and become a positive thinker, though many people certainly try. It's not that easy. You learn to look at your thoughts from many different perspectives—negatively, positively and neutrally—as you consider new solutions and conclusions.

3. EXAMINING YOUR BELIEFS. Some thoughts pop up without your control, almost automatically. These thoughts are based on deeply held beliefs about yourself and about others. These thoughts may annoy you that you are even thinking them. For example, if you believe that "most people are out for themselves," you'll hear a constant stream of negative thoughts whenever you find yourself in a situation that confirms this view. Some of these beliefs are accurate, but some are not. You will learn how to tell the difference and replace unrealistic, unfounded beliefs with more accurate ones that will fuel balanced thinking and better moods.

4. CHANGING YOUR BEHAVIOR. You might be wondering, "What if my thoughts *are* justified? What if people truly *are* treating me badly?" That's where changing your behavior comes in. In addition to changing your thoughts, you will also work at changing the behaviors that kindle your negative thoughts and moods. Just changing your thoughts doesn't make your doctor treat you with more respect, for example. However, changing your deeply held core belief from "I can't do anything about my health" to "My health is under my control" could ignite the motivation to find a new doctor.

HOW TO PRACTICE COGNITIVE BEHAVIOR THERAPY

Getting in touch with your habitual moods, feelings, thoughts, beliefs, and behavior takes some work. Like a detective, you need to keep a written record of your observations so that you can act on them systematically. As you complete the six steps for learning cognitive behavior therapy, you will begin to separate your inner, nonbiased self from the more biased and not-as-trustworthy feelings and automatic thoughts that are currently controlling your inner and outer worlds. In order to do this, you must make notes. You can make these notes either in the planner in Chapter 9 or in a separate notebook.

Your first step is getting in touch with your moods and feelings. Then you'll move on to examine your thoughts, then your beliefs, and, by week 6, your behaviors. Read through the explanations for weeks 1 though 6, which follow, before you attempt the exercises so that you understand the process. Then move on to Chapter 9 and your six-week planner, which will walk you through each step of the cognitive behavior therapy technique, one day at a time. This six-week planner contains logs, reflective questions, and exercises to help you accomplish each goal, and it tells you when to reread certain sections of the chapter to complete certain exercises. I recommend that you buy a small notebook that you can carry and use as a diary. In it, you can write down thoughts and moods as they come up, and record the answers to the questions that are in the weekly planner.

Let's get started.

Week 1: Getting in Touch with Your Moods and Feelings

Your first step in lifting depression, controlling anger, and reducing anxiety lies in noticing the earliest signs of such negative moods. Then you can pinpoint the circumstances surrounding your moods, the thoughts and beliefs that lead to them, and the behaviors that stem from them. This may sound easy, but it isn't.

Many of us are in touch with our moods enough to describe them as "good" or "bad," but in order to change your moods, you must be able to describe them more specifically. For example, if you are feeling "bad," does that mean that you are angry, sad, frustrated, anxious, irritated, or something else? If you are feeling "good," does that mean that you are happy, peaceful, content, joyful, excited, or something else?

In addition to pinpointing your exact mood, you will learn to sense moods as they arise. This will help you to link your moods to particular situations and thoughts that may have triggered them.

To start, think back over your past week. Try to pinpoint times when you may have felt a particular mood. If you have trouble doing this, try to identify uncomfortable bodily reactions. Do you remember your hands sweating for "no reason"? Do you remember your heart pounding, feeling hot in the face, feeling tension in your muscles, or noticing that you had clenched fists? Think back to your behavior. Did you cancel going out and decide to spend the day in bed? Did you throw a book across the room? Did you feel so rattled that you couldn't think straight?

What was that mood? Use a single word to describe it, and write it down in your notebook. You should be able to describe your mood with one word. If it takes more than one word, you may instead be describing the thought that led to the mood. If you have trouble, consult the "Common Moods" box.

Once you pinpoint a mood, recall the situation that surrounded it. What were you doing just before you felt that way? Who were you with? What were you talking about? Write this down.

You may begin to feel like a detective who is uncovering the facts of the situation. Look for all of the evidence surrounding your mood. Write down all the facts you can remember in the half-hour surrounding the mood, listing the who, what, where, and when of the situation. Write down as many details as possible, and be as specific as possible. Once you are done, you should have some additional facts that help you understand the cause of your mood. Let's say you notice that you are angry early one morning. To describe the situation, you would write, "I walked into the kitchen to make breakfast. A pile of dishes was in the sink and I couldn't find a single clean bowl. I ended up washing all the dishes before making breakfast. When I looked at my watch and realized I was late for work, I felt angry."

In coming weeks, you'll learn how to find out more facts to understand your moods. For now, simply concentrate on noticing your moods and the surrounding situation as they unfold. In Chapter 9, your planner will prompt you to jot down your moods during week 1. Write in your planner whenever you feel sad, irritable, depressed, angry, or negative in any way. Your goal is to notice at least one mood each day during week 1. By week 2, when you look back over your planner entries, each day should have something written down.

COMMON MOODS

Here are some common moods that all of us feel on a regular basis:

> Love
> Excitement
> Contentment
> Sadness
> Happiness
> Anger
> Worry
> Fear
> Guilt
> Shame
> Irritation
> Frustration
> Humiliation
> Panic
> Nervousness
> Rage
> Disgust
> Pride

Week 2: Getting in Touch with Your Thoughts

After you're in better touch with your moods and the situations that seem to trigger them, it's time to start tracking the automatic thoughts that might be leading to your moods.

At any given moment, a constant stream of thoughts is running through your mind. To hear it, sit quietly for a few moments right now and notice the mental chatter. Do nothing else but monitor your thoughts. You'll probably be surprised by some of the mundane things that pop up. You'll also be surprised to see how hard it is to stop thoughts from popping up. It can seem as if the brain truly does have a mind of its own.

It takes a great deal of concentration to slow down and stop your thoughts. When your child comes home with a bad report card and you think, "She's never going to get anywhere in life," that's an automatic thought. That automatic thought might lead to a stream of other thoughts such as, "Can't this kid do anything right? Isn't it bad enough that I've got to work and clean the house and help the kids with their homework and test my blood sugar and watch my diet? Can't she just come home with a decent report card? Is that too much to ask?" With such negative thoughts, anyone would feel sad or angry.

For week 2 you will concentrate on pinpointing thoughts that lead to certain moods. To get started, look back over your planner entries from week 1. Mentally bring yourself back to a few of the situations. Can you remember what was running through your mind before you felt a particular mood? If so, write it down in your notebook.

Notice what was going through your mind when you felt a certain way in a certain situation. Write down words, phrases, or images that you thought just before you were feeling that emotion or as you feel it. It might even be a memory of something that happened to you earlier in life.

For week 2, you will keep track of your moods *and* your thoughts. Be particularly on the lookout for negative, self-defeating, or cynical mind chatter, such as, "I'm no good," "People always let me down," or "I can't get a break." If you're anxious, you'll look for catastrophic thoughts; if you're hostile, you'll look for cynical thoughts about yourself, others, and the world in general; and if you're depressed, you'll look for self-defeating thoughts.

Monitor your thoughts throughout the day, and jot down key moods and thoughts. Whenever you catch yourself thinking negatively, write it down, along with the time and situation and your mood. Make sure to identify the who, what, where, when, and why of each situation. Write down exactly what your thoughts are, no matter how embarrassing. No one is going to see this, so don't edit yourself. Also be sure to write down only the thoughts that occurred to you at that moment, not thoughts that came to you afterward. Your thoughts will help you make sense of your moods, particularly moods that seem unrelated to your situation.

Write out your thoughts in complete sentences. As a general rule of thumb, if you think you can describe a thought in one word, you are probably instead describing your mood. Sometimes your thoughts will be verbal; at other times, your thoughts may come to you in visions or memories. Write down anything that comes into your head that puts you in a negative mood.

To help you along, consult the "Pinpointing Thoughts" box for help in describing your thoughts. After you write down your thoughts, look them over. Which seem most related to your mood? Circle them. Your most influential thoughts are the ones that could make you feel a negative mood even without the triggering situation.

At first, you may need to take your notebook with you and sit down and do this exercise as soon as you feel a mood so that you can remember your thoughts. The more you do this exercise, you will automatically notice your thoughts and feelings and be able to remember them. These words or images go through your mind somewhat quickly. It will take a little practice to learn to catch them.

PINPOINTING THOUGHTS

As you write about your thoughts, ask yourself:

• What was I thinking just before I felt this mood?
• What images did I see just before a negative mood set in?
• What was I daydreaming about just before noticing a negative mood?
• What memories were triggered when I felt a negative mood?

Week 3: Testing Your Thoughts

Now that you've pinpointed some of the thoughts that may be triggering your moods, it's time to test them for accuracy. Some of your thoughts may be completely valid; some may not. Your mood will shift as you uncover evidence that counters the validity of your thoughts and feelings. To sort out the accurate thoughts from the flawed ones, you'll conduct an experiment.

Continue to keep your mood and thought journal for week 3 as described in your planner in Chapter 9, again writing down the thoughts and situations surrounding your negative moods. This week, however, you will take the exercise one step further: begin to examine those thoughts from different angles.

Your thoughts may suffer from any of the following types of dysfunctional thinking:

• **ALL-OR-NOTHING THINKING.** These thoughts describe you, others, and the world in black-and-white terms with no room for a gray middle ground. For example, if your boss mistreats you once at work, your all-or-nothing thoughts may tell you, "She's completely evil" or "She hates me." If your doctor tells you that your average blood sugar is higher than normal, all-or-nothing thoughts may tell you, "It doesn't matter what I do. My diabetes will always be out of control."

• **OVERLY GENERAL THINKING.** Similar to all-or-nothing thoughts, these messages omit qualifiers such as *most, sometimes, rarely,* and *often.* Instead, your thoughts tend to include the word *always.* For example, instead of thinking, "I feel tired when I don't get enough sleep," you might think, "I always feel tired."

• MENTAL FILTERING. It's almost as if your thoughts run through a filter that siphons off all of the positive evidence in yourself, other people, and the rest of the world in general before they enter your consciousness.

• MENTAL REFEREEING. Similar to filtered thoughts, these thoughts act as the devil's advocate to any positive thoughts that might slip into your consciousness. For example, if someone compliments a coworker on a job well done, your internal referee may find a way to discount and disqualify the positive information so that you can maintain your belief that this coworker never seems to measure up to expectations.

• MIND READING. These thoughts assume negative things about other people and the future that are impossible to know. For example, if your mother calls at the last minute to tell you that she can't baby-sit your kids tonight as she promised, your mind-reading thoughts might tell you, "She's mad that I didn't call her this morning, and now she's trying to get back at me." Or if your doctor walks into the office with a frown on her face, you might think, "Oh, she's got terrible news for me."

• CATASTROPHIZING. These thoughts exaggerate negative situations and underestimate positive ones. For example, if you make a mistake at work, your catastrophic thoughts might tell you that you will be fired.

• EMOTIONAL THINKING. These thoughts stem from negative moods. When you feel bad or angry, your thoughts work to justify your mood. For example, instead of questioning your anger, you let emotional thoughts justify lashing out at someone.

• "SHOULD" THINKING. Some funny person who will probably forever remain anonymous once remarked, "No one likes to be should upon." "Should" thoughts either make you feel guilty ("I should have found the energy to do that") or make you angry or disappointed with someone else ("My kids should be old enough to not do this anymore").

• LABELING. These thoughts create a self-fulfilling prophecy. You label yourself a hothead and therefore give yourself permission to blow up at people. You label someone else irresponsible and therefore are quick to get angry when he lets you down.

As you write down your thoughts in week 3, you will test them against these flawed ways of thinking. You will also challenge your thoughts by asking yourself:

- Is there any evidence that supports these thoughts?
- Is there any evidence that does not support my thoughts?
- Have I jumped to conclusions?
- Am I shouldering too much blame?
- Did I use any of the flawed thought processes?
- If a good friend knew about these thoughts, what would she or he tell me?
- Are there any things that I am ignoring that could discount these thoughts?
- Is there another way to see this situation?

Once a day, you will list your moods and rate them, write down the situations surrounding them, and the thoughts that ran through your mind. You will also begin to rate your thoughts on a scale of 1 to 10 according to how much you believe them. A rating of 1 means you don't believe it at all, and a 10 means you believe it 100 percent. Analyze your thoughts, and then again rate them on a scale from 1 to 10. Don't be surprised if your rating changes. Again, keep notes on this in your planner or notebook.

Week 4: Pinpointing Your Beliefs

Thoughts are the verbal and visual messages that run through your mind; your assumptions and beliefs run much deeper. Now that you're in better touch with your moods and thoughts, it's time to uncover the deeply held beliefs that lead to your negative automatic thoughts and moods. Examining and challenging these beliefs is the key to stopping self-defeating thoughts.

In many cases, these beliefs revolve around "if-then" and "should" assumptions. For instance, you may assume that you should be nice to your children all of the time or that you must work twelve hours a day to be successful. Core beliefs run even deeper than your assumptions. These are how you generally see yourself, others, and the rest of the world. For example, a core belief about yourself might be, "I am worthless"; one about others might be, "She's not dependable"; and one about the world, "People can't be trusted." Core beliefs are absolute. They have no qualifiers.

Getting at these assumptions and beliefs will help slow the flow of negative thoughts into your head. Because you formed many of your assumptions and beliefs during childhood and early adulthood, they will be harder to confront and replace than your everyday thoughts. Often your beliefs stem from information you received about the world from an early age. For example, if you grew up in a dysfunctional home with abusive parents, you may never have felt safe or had someone you could trust early in life. As a result, you may have grown up believing, "I must protect myself from others" or, "The only person who watches out for me is me."

We learn beliefs from the behavior and verbal messages that were modeled for us early in life. Just as you may share many of your political beliefs with your parents, you may also discover that your deep internal beliefs that lead you to anger, depression, or anxiety came from comments your parents made over and over again when you were young.

No matter where these beliefs came from, it's time to face them, sift out the negative and inaccurate ones, and replace them with more realistic and positive beliefs. It's like switching over from something that you're comfortable with to something new that you're not. For example, when you switched from a VCR to a DVD player, the switch may at first have seemed frustrating. You may have felt attached to your old video collection. The DVD player may have seemed too complicated to operate. But after some time, you broke in the DVD and you trained yourself and your mind to understand it. Now you probably wouldn't want to switch back because the quality on the DVD is so much better.

It's the same with developing new beliefs. At first you will feel uncomfortable and may not even fully believe in the process. Over time, however, as your thinking changes, you'll see that the new way is better and you won't be able to understand how you could have stuck with your old beliefs for so long.

You'll start by looking over the entries you made in your planner or notebook for the past few weeks. Is there a common theme to your thoughts? Do you have the same thoughts over and over? What beliefs about yourself or others might be leading to those thoughts? Ask yourself:

- What does this thought say about me?
- What does this thought mean about my life?
- What does this thought mean about the person it's directed toward?
- What does this thought say about the world in general?

Answering these questions will help you arrive at some of your deeply held beliefs. For example, let's say that when you look over your notebook entries, you notice that you often found yourself thinking, "I can't do it all." To answer the question, "What does this thought say about me?" you might write, "I'm incompetent." That's an assumption about yourself that may or may not be true. Here's another example. Let's say you noticed yourself thinking, "Cheryl's health has never been a problem for her, but I have diabetes." When you examine, "What does this thought say about Cheryl?" you might write, "Cheryl has it easy." That may or may not be true.

Once you pinpoint your negative beliefs, you will then replace them with more accurate, positive beliefs. Each day for week 4, you will examine one belief, looking for evidence during the day that either confirms or contradicts it. You might start by finding just one or two facts a day. If that feels easy, move on to finding three or four. Eventually you want to write down every bit of evidence that you can find either for or against your beliefs.

For example, let's go back to the belief that Cheryl has it easy. When you gather evidence, you might realize that Cheryl's mother has been sick for a long time, that she's a single mother raising three children, and that she long ago gave up her dream of getting a college education. You may decide that Cheryl doesn't have it so easy after all.

Week 5: Replacing Your Beliefs and Thoughts

Now that you know that some of your beliefs and automatic thoughts aren't completely true, it's time to come up with valid ones. This week, you will take your old flawed beliefs and rewrite them into more accurate, positive views of yourself, others, and the rest of the world. For example, if you believe, "Diabetes has ruined my life," you might want to revise that to be, "Diabetes has certainly made my life harder, but not impossible."

Coming up with alternate beliefs is only half the battle. You must actually believe these new statements for them to change your automatic thoughts and eventually your moods. To do that, you will again gather evidence, this time looking for facts that support your new way of thinking.

Each day during week 5, you will examine one old belief that you identified as flawed from the week before. Next to that belief, you will write at least one alternate belief or assumption. Before testing that new alternate belief, rate its believability on a scale from 1 to 10, with one being "very hard to believe" and 10 being "completely believable."

You might find it easier to do some of this as homework on the first day of week 5, picking six beliefs, listing them in the space provided in the days to come, and then rating them. That way, each day you need only look at your notes to find the belief to test and the evidence to gather. At first, finding evidence that supports your new beliefs may feel difficult. Eventually, the process becomes easier.

As you change your beliefs, you'll begin to notice automatically when negative or destructive thoughts pop up, sense that they are not completely accurate, and stop them or rewrite them before they can trigger a bad mood. Eventually, those negative thoughts will pop up less often.

Week 6: Changing Your Reactions

Once you have a handle on your moods, thoughts, and beliefs, it's time to take a look at your reactions. Even though your anger, frustration, sadness, or disappointment may be justified, that doesn't mean you still must respond with an inappropriate reaction of lashing out, yelling, throwing objects, locking yourself in your room, or inflicting the silent treatment.

Think of a problem or situation where you have learned that your reactions are not logical. For instance, while standing in line at the supermarket, the person in front of you decides he forgot something and goes to get it, leaving the other items on the counter. The checkout person has to stop what she is doing. There is nothing you can do in this situation, but the people involved in it are not necessarily stupid or inconsiderate. Instead of getting angry and tense, focus on something else, like the magazine rack next to the checkout counter. By the time you finish reading an article, chances are the person in front of you will have come back, and the checkout process will proceed.

You can find a nonviolent solution to any situation. You need only think of many possible solutions—even silly ones. Your goal is to solve the problem and improve the situation, not to get even. Don't discount any solution just yet. Allow the creative side of your brain to operate unfettered, coming up with one possible solution after another.

If you have trouble coming up with ideas, try the following:

- Think back over your life. Have you come across this issue or problem before? If so, how did you respond? Did any of those responses help improve the situation? Did any make the situation worse?
- Ask a close friend or family member for help. Talk over your problem, and ask the friend or family member what she or he would do in the same situation.
- If you don't feel comfortable talking about the problem with someone you know, go on-line. Search for a chatroom or discussion board related to the problem you are experiencing. If

you already belong to a discussion list, post your problem, and ask others for ideas.

• Check to see if automatic thoughts are getting in your way. Thoughts such as, "I'm not good enough" or even "This is stupid," may be causing you to discount possible solutions.

After you have thought up possible solutions, examine each. Imagine yourself enacting each solution, and then imagine what might happen next. After weighing your pros and cons, select the solution that seems most promising and poses the least risk for generating negative results.

Once you've arrived at a solution, do it. Then, assess how well things went. If your solution failed to work or you encountered unanticipated negative results, don't worry. Just look at it as a learning experience, and start the process over again.

CHECKLIST FOR SOLVING PROBLEMS

If you are having trouble with a particular person or situation and want to change it, follow this process:

1. Recognize the problem. What is it?
2. Define it. What is causing the problem?
3. Think of many different solutions.
4. Pick the solution that seems as if it will work the best.
5. Try it, and then examine the results.

THE POWER OF SUPPORT

Supportive people take the sting out of life. Study after study shows that people who have numerous close social ties not only tend to live longer and feel better emotionally, they are also better able to stick to exercise programs, lose weight, and generally make important changes in their lives. Having support as you go through the program in this book will help you too. Resist the urge to do this alone, particularly if you scored high on the depression or hostility tests in Chapter 6. Many people, particularly those who are hostile or depressed, have trouble reaching out to others. If this were easy, you'd already have a strong social network, right? Hostile types believe that others are untrustworthy and out for themselves. Depressed people feel there's no way others could possibly love them.

Other people can help you talk through your thoughts, release steam, and generally comfort you. They can help you brainstorm solutions to your problems, examine flawed ways of thinking, and just generally be there to help you face the ups and downs of life. Your support network can include doctors, friends, family, church members, clergy, and counselors. You need people who can give you advice, help reduce pressure by doing errands and chores, or just listen and be there for you. You'll need at least three different types of support:

- A health supporter—someone who helps ease the burden of diabetes by giving you information and advice.
- A chore supporter—someone who helps ease the burden of diabetes by doing tasks and helping you to get everything done. This person is also someone you can call in an emergency.
- An emotional supporter—someone who listens, helps you overcome bad moods, helps build up your confidence, and generally makes you feel good.

As a first step in establishing your support team, write down beliefs that may be holding you back from forming better connections with others. For example, do you believe that if you ask others for help, they will think that you are weak, can't take care of yourself, or can't solve your own problems? Do you feel that asking for help is asking for too much and that competent people can get through life without help? Do you think that asking for help means that others will take advantage of you, talk down to you, use you, misguide you, or reveal your secrets to others? Do you think you are already a burden to others as it is? Do you feel that you are already unlovable and that no one in his or her right mind would want to help you?

Examine those beliefs with the same cognitive behavior therapy process outlined in this six-week program. Once you've gotten over your emotional roadblock, think of other people who can help fill each role for you. Then talk to each one and ask for his or her help.

GETTING PROFESSIONAL HELP

Cognitive behavior therapy is a form of psychotherapy. If you feel that you are spinning your wheels and just can't get yourself to change the way you see and react to situations, I recommend that you try a few sessions with a well-trained cognitive behavior therapist who can help guide you and coach you through the changes that you need to make. If you are depressed and you feel that the self-help techniques aren't working, you must see a therapist. I have provided a variety of resources in Chapter 13 to help you contact a qualified person.

9

Putting It All Together

Your Step-by-Step Six-Week Planner

THIS chapter will help you keep track of your progress as you learn progressive muscle relaxation and cognitive behavior therapy. The day-by-day tips, questions, and checklists will help you learn one technique or both, allowing you to create a customized six-week mind-body program that addresses your specific psychological needs.

If you scored low in hostility and depression in the quizzes, you may focus just on progressive muscle relaxation. If you scored low for stress but high for depression or hostility, you may focus just on cognitive behavior therapy. If you scored high for stress and depression or hostility, tackle both the progressive muscle relaxation and cognitive behavior therapy techniques together. For each day, every aspect of the program is clearly marked, so you can choose which exercises to focus on for that day.

By the end of the program, you'll feel less stress, anxiety, and depression. If you do not notice results right away, be patient. You may simply need to practice a little longer. Focus on each small success along your journey to a healthier, calmer mind. You should also see changes in your blood sugar control within these six weeks, but it can take longer for such physical changes to occur. This doesn't mean the program isn't working. Be patient, and stay the course. Within six months you should notice significant changes in your physical health.

Six weeks is the usual amount of time it takes to learn these new mental habits and practice them consistently. By the end of that time, the techniques will feel natural to you. After the initial six weeks, these actions will start becoming a habit. Each of the seventy-four pages starting on page 122 contains specific instructions on how to progress. I've included numerous ways to help you keep track of your "homework," as well as reflective questions and a good amount of space to write your answers. You may prefer to use a separate notebook rather than writing in this book.

Before you get started, assess your condition by answering the questions that follow. These answers will help you to gauge your progress and fuel your motivation to stick with your program. Write your answers below or in your notebook.

Assessing Your Condition

According to the stages of change model described in Chapter 6, I'm at this stage: _____

My fasting blood sugar level is _____.

According to the "Test Your Stress Response" questions on page 69, stress is a problem for me. _____

According to the "Test Your Depression Level" quiz on pages 70 to 71, depression is a problem for me. _____

According to the "Test Your Hostility Level" quiz on page 71, hostility is a problem for me. _____

I feel stressed or anxious (a) nearly every day, (b) most days, (c) once a week, (d) every once in a while, (e) rarely. _____

I feel sad or depressed (a) nearly every day, (b) most days, (c) once a week, (d) every once in a while, (e) rarely. _____

I feel angry (a) nearly every day, (b) most days, (c) once a week, (d) every once in a while, (e) rarely. _____

I feel a sense of deep relaxation and inner peace (a) nearly every day, (b) most days, (c) once a week, (d) every once in a while, (e) rarely. _____

Save your answers to these questions so that you can refer to them after six weeks and then again after six months. They will help you see how much progress you've made. All too often, positive changes in health and emotional well-being occur so gradually that we fail to notice and acknowledge them. This will help you celebrate each success along your Mind-Body Diabetes Revolution journey.

Be sure you have read Chapters 7 and 8 before embarking on this six-week journey. Those chapters provide the framework that you will use for the next forty-two days. During each day of the next six weeks, I'll ask you to reread certain sections of those chapters to refamiliarize yourself with the material.

Week 1

Every now and then go away, have a little relaxation, for when you come back to your work your judgment will be surer. Go some distance away because then the work appears smaller and more of it can be taken in at a glance and a lack of harmony and proportion is more readily seen.

—Leonardo da Vinci

This week in your progressive muscle relaxation segment, you'll spend about 20 minutes two times a day doing progressive muscle relaxation, based on script 1 in Chapter 7. Before and after each session, you will rate your tension level on a scale of 1 to 10, with 1 feeling very calm and 10 feeling extremely anxious. Make sure that you have created a tape to listen to, purchased the CD, or have someone to read the script to you. For your cognitive behavior therapy segment, you will focus on noticing your moods and the situations that surround them. Reread pages 105 to 107 in Chapter 8 to familiarize yourself with this process and do the suggested homework exercises before you start off your week.

Day 1

A journey of a thousand miles begins with but a single step.

—Chinese proverb

PROGRESSIVE MUSCLE RELAXATION

Complete two 20-minute relaxation sessions:

Yes, I completed session 1: _____
Yes, I completed session 2: _____

Before and after each session, rate your tension level on a scale from 1 to 10:

Session 1: My tension level before relaxation: _____
Session 1: My tension level after relaxation: _____
Session 2: My tension level before relaxation: _____
Session 2: My tension level after relaxation: _____

COGNITIVE BEHAVIOR THERAPY

Think back over your day. Write down any strong moods that you noticed. Rank your moods in intensity on a scale from 1 to 10 (1 equals neutral and 10 equals the strongest mood you've ever felt). Then describe the surrounding situation—who you were with, what you were doing, what you were talking about, and so on:

My mood: _____
My mood's intensity (1 to 10): _____
The situation (who, what, where, when):

TODAY'S TIP

Often we blame others and don't take responsibility for the behavior that stems from our own negative emotions. Instead of automatically placing the blame on others, look at a situation from all angles and every viewpoint. Write down the names of each person involved, and list how each contributed to the encounter. Rank each person's responsibility in creating your mood. You'll see that you are also responsible for your moods and reactions. After you own up to your share of the responsibility, ask yourself whether you should make amends.

Day 2

Life is what happens to us while we are making other plans

—*John Lennon*

PROGRESSIVE MUSCLE RELAXATION

Complete two 20-minute relaxation sessions:

Yes, I completed session 1: ___
Yes, I completed session 2: ___

Before and after each session, rate your tension level on a scale from 1 to 10:

Session 1: My tension level before relaxation: ____
Session 1: My tension level after relaxation: ____
Session 2: My tension level before relaxation: ____
Session 2: My tension level after relaxation: ____

COGNITIVE BEHAVIOR THERAPY

Think back over your day. Write down any strong moods that you noticed. Rank your moods in intensity on a scale from 1 to 10. Then describe the surrounding situation—who you were with, what you were doing, what you were talking about, and so on:

My mood: ____
My mood's intensity (1 to 10): ____
The situation:

TODAY'S TIP

When you are depressed and turning anger inward against yourself, it often helps to talk to someone else about what's going on inside your head. Talk to a friend or someone else you trust about the situation. Explain your guilt or shame and the surrounding circumstances. Often just talking about it and getting your secret off your chest will lift a weight off your shoulders. Also, your friend will probably tell you that you're being too hard on yourself.

Day 3

People are as happy as they make up their minds to be.

—*Abe Lincoln*

PROGRESSIVE MUSCLE RELAXATION

Complete two 20-minute relaxation sessions:

Yes, I completed session 1: ___
Yes, I completed session 2: ___

Before and after each session, rate your tension level on a scale from 1 to 10:

Session 1: My tension level before relaxation: ____
Session 1: My tension level after relaxation: ____
Session 2: My tension level before relaxation: ____
Session 2: My tension level after relaxation: ____

COGNITIVE BEHAVIOR THERAPY

Think back over your day. Write down any strong moods that you noticed. Rank your moods in intensity on a scale from 1 to 10. Then describe the surrounding situation—who you were with, what you were doing, what you were talking about, and so on:

My mood: ____
My mood's intensity (1 to 10): ____

The situation:

TODAY'S TIP
If you hurt someone because of your anger, apologize to that person. Find the courage to face him or her and try to fix the damage.

Day 4
The best way to cheer yourself up is to try to cheer somebody else up.

—*Mark Twain*

PROGRESSIVE MUSCLE RELAXATION
Complete two 20-minute relaxation sessions:

Yes, I completed session 1: ___
Yes, I completed session 2: ___

Before and after each session, rate your tension level on a scale from 1 to 10:

Session 1: My tension level before relaxation: ____
Session 1: My tension level after relaxation: ____
Session 2: My tension level before relaxation: ____
Session 2: My tension level after relaxation: ____

COGNITIVE BEHAVIOR THERAPY
Think back over your day. Write down any strong moods that you noticed. Rank your moods in intensity on a scale from 1 to 10. Then describe the surrounding situation—including who you were with, what you were doing, what you were talking about, and so on:

My mood: ____
My mood's intensity (1 to 10): ____
The situation:

TODAY'S TIP

The more close relationships you have, the better you will feel. Similarly, if you have many toxic relationships, it will be tough to recover from depression, hostility, or stress. As you progress along the program, maximize your contact with positive people who support your efforts and comfort you in times of stress. When possible, minimize your contact with negative people who ignore your needs and tend to trigger your negative moods.

Day 5

You gain strength, courage and confidence by every experience in which you really stop to look fear in the face. You are able to say to yourself, "I have lived through this horror. I can take the next thing that comes along." You must do the thing you think you cannot do.

—*Eleanor Roosevelt*

PROGRESSIVE MUSCLE RELAXATION

Complete two 20-minute relaxation sessions:

Yes, I completed session 1: ___
Yes, I completed session 2: ___

Before and after each session, rate your tension level on a scale from 1 to 10:

Session 1: My tension level before relaxation: ____
Session 1: My tension level after relaxation: ____
Session 2: My tension level before relaxation: ____
Session 2: My tension level after relaxation: ____

COGNITIVE BEHAVIOR THERAPY

Think back over your day. Write down any strong moods that you noticed. Rank your moods in intensity on a scale from 1 to 10. Then describe the surrounding situation—who you were with, what you were doing, what you were talking about, and so on:

My mood: ____
My mood's intensity: (1 to 10) ____
The situation:

TODAY'S TIP

Regular exercise helps maximize levels of soothing brain chemicals, which lifts depression and calms stress and anger. If you keep an activity log, you'll probably notice that you are most irritable or depressed on the days or weeks that you are most sedentary. When you exercise, resist the urge to make it a competition. This is for your enjoyment. Don't beat yourself up if you miss a session.

Day 6

We all live in suspense, from day to day, from hour to hour; in other words, we are the hero of our own story.

—*Mary McCarthy, writer*

Progressive Muscle Relaxation

Complete two 20-minute relaxation sessions:

Yes, I completed session 1: ___
Yes, I completed session 2: ___

Before and after each session, rate your tension level on a scale from 1 to 10:

Session 1: My tension level before relaxation: ____
Session 1: My tension level after relaxation: ____
Session 2: My tension level before relaxation: ____
Session 2: My tension level after relaxation: ____

Cognitive Behavior Therapy

Think back over your day. Write down any strong moods that you noticed. Rank your moods in intensity on a scale from 1 to 10. Then describe the surrounding situation—who you were with, what you were doing, what you were talking about, and so on:

My mood: ____
My mood's intensity (1 to 10): ____
The situation:

Today's Tip

Challenge your moods and thoughts. When you catch yourself catastrophizing or thinking negatively, ask yourself, "What then? How bad could this be? What's the worst thing that can happen?" Put your thoughts, mood, and the situation in perspective by imagining yourself looking back on the situation

five years from now. Five years from now, will you care this
deeply?

Day 7

You are the architect of your personal experience.

—*Shirley MacLaine*

PROGRESSIVE MUSCLE RELAXATION
Complete two 20-minute relaxation sessions:

Yes, I completed session 1: ___
Yes, I completed session 2: ___

Before and after each session, rate your tension level on a
scale from 1 to 10:

Session 1: My tension level before relaxation: ____
Session 1: My tension level after relaxation: ____
Session 2: My tension level before relaxation: ____
Session 2: My tension level after relaxation: ____

COGNITIVE BEHAVIOR THERAPY
Think back over your day. Write down any strong moods that
you noticed. Rank your moods in intensity on a scale from 1 to
10. Then describe the surrounding situation—who you were
with, what you were doing, what you were talking about, and so
on:

My mood: ____
My mood's intensity (1 to 10): ____
The situation:

Look back over your week. Do you notice a pattern to your moods and situations? If so, write down some thoughts here:

Today's Tip

Review your planner entries each week, and look for patterns. Try to see what your entries can teach you about yourself. Look for common themes in situations, thoughts, moods, and beliefs. Summarize them on a sheet of paper. When you look back at situations, you may feel guilty or ashamed at your reactions to them. Sometimes, however, your reactions are right on target, and this exercise will help you to see that.

Week 2

Each problem that I solved became a rule which served afterwards to solve other problems.

—René Descartes, philosopher

For progressive muscle relaxation this week, you will learn how to relax without first tensing your muscles. Once you can mentally coax your muscles to relax, you'll be able to use progressive muscle relaxation in any situation when you find yourself tense—without anyone else knowing what you are doing.

For cognitive behavior therapy this week, you will begin to pinpoint the thoughts that lead to certain moods. Reread this section under "Week 2" in Chapter 8 before getting started, making sure to complete the suggested exercises. Carry a notebook or journal with you this week to record your thoughts so that you can remember them later.

Day 8

I don't want to be a passenger in my own life.

—Diane Ackerman, poet and essayist

Progressive Muscle Relaxation

Complete two 20-minute relaxation sessions—one with progressive muscle relaxation script 1 and one with progressive muscle relaxation script 2:

Yes, I completed session 1: ___
Yes, I completed session 2: ___

Before and after each session, rate your tension level on a scale from 1 to 10:

Session 1: My tension level before relaxation: ____
Session 1: My tension level after relaxation: ____
Session 2: My tension level before relaxation: ____
Session 2: My tension level after relaxation: ____

Cognitive Behavior Therapy

Whenever you notice yourself in a bad mood, try to catch the thoughts that run through your head:

My mood: ____
My mood's intensity (1 to 10): ____
The situation:

My thoughts just before the mood set in:

TODAY'S TIP
Don't expect others to read your mind. For example, tell your spouse that your anniversary is coming up and that you expect to be treated to a romantic dinner. Just as you can't know the inner needs of others, they can't know yours unless you tell them.

Day 9
As one goes through life one learns that if you don't paddle your own canoe, you don't move.
—*Katharine Hepburn*

PROGRESSIVE MUSCLE RELAXATION
Complete two 20-minute relaxation sessions—one with progressive muscle relaxation script 1 and one with progressive muscle relaxation script 2:

Yes, I completed session 1: ___
Yes, I completed session 2: ___

Before and after each session, rate your tension level on a scale from 1 to 10:

Session 1: My tension level before relaxation: ____
Session 1: My tension level after relaxation: ____
Session 2: My tension level before relaxation: ____
Session 2: My tension level after relaxation: ____

COGNITIVE BEHAVIOR THERAPY
Whenever you notice yourself in a bad mood, try to catch the thoughts that run through your head:

My mood: ____
My mood's intensity (1 to 10): ____
The situation:

My thoughts just before the mood set in:

TODAY'S TIP

If you knew you were going to die tomorrow, would you spend today ranting about your boss, yelling at your neighbor, moaning about the mail carrier, or stressed about picking up after your kids? Probably not. Life is a series of moments linked together by you and your memories. Make each moment count.

Day 10

If we don't change, we don't grow. If we don't grow, we are not really living.

—Gail Sheehy, author

PROGRESSIVE MUSCLE RELAXATION

Complete two 20-minute relaxation sessions—one with progressive muscle relaxation script 1 and one with progressive muscle relaxation script 2:

Yes, I completed session 1: ____
Yes, I completed session 2: ____

Before and after each session, rate your tension level on a scale from 1 to 10:

Session 1: My tension level before relaxation: ____
Session 1: My tension level after relaxation: ____
Session 2: My tension level before relaxation: ____
Session 2: My tension level after relaxation: ____

COGNITIVE BEHAVIOR THERAPY

Whenever you notice yourself in a bad mood, try to catch the thoughts that run through your head:

My mood: ____
My mood's intensity (1 to 10): ____
The situation:

My thoughts just before the mood set in:

TODAY'S TIP

Do you feel more comfortable listening or talking? If you are depressed, the answer is probably listening. If you scored high for hostility in Chapter 6, the answer is probably talking. If you are having trouble deciding, ask the question in reverse: Which makes you more uncomfortable—listening or talking? Once you arrive at your answer, practice whichever of the two you find more difficult.

Day 11

Sometimes I lie awake at night, and I ask, "Where have I gone wrong?" Then a voice says to me, "This is going to take more than one night."

—*Charlie Brown*

PROGRESSIVE MUSCLE RELAXATION

Complete two 20-minute relaxation sessions—one with progressive muscle relaxation script 1 and one with progressive muscle relaxation script 2:

Yes, I completed session 1: _____
Yes, I completed session 2: _____

Before and after each session, rate your tension level on a scale from 1 to 10:

Session 1: My tension level before relaxation: _____
Session 1: My tension level after relaxation: _____
Session 2: My tension level before relaxation: _____
Session 2: My tension level after relaxation: _____

COGNITIVE BEHAVIOR THERAPY

Whenever you notice yourself in a bad mood, try to catch the thoughts that run through your head:

My mood: _____
My mood's intensity (1 to 10): _____
The situation:

My thoughts just before the mood set in:

TODAY'S TIP

Helping another person in need will help you feel better about yourself and about others and the rest of the world. Sign up for a regular volunteer activity, such as driving a Meals on Wheels route, ladling out soup at a homeless shelter, or tutoring a child or adult at a community center. You can find social outreach programs through your religious establishment or in the Yellow Pages.

Day 12
I was always looking outside myself for strength and confidence but it comes from within. It is there all the time.
                                                        —*Anna Freud*

PROGRESSIVE MUSCLE RELAXATION
Complete two 20-minute relaxation sessions, one with progressive muscle relaxation script 1 and one with progressive muscle relaxation script 2:

Yes, I completed session 1: _____
Yes, I completed session 2: _____

Before and after each session, rate your tension level on a scale from 1 to 10:

Session 1: My tension level before relaxation: _____
Session 1: My tension level after relaxation: _____
Session 2: My tension level before relaxation: _____
Session 2: My tension level after relaxation: _____

COGNITIVE BEHAVIOR THERAPY
Whenever you notice yourself in a bad mood, try to catch the thoughts that run through your head:

My mood: _____
My mood's intensity (1 to 10): _____
The situation:

My thoughts just before the mood set in:

Today's Tip

Examining your thoughts and changing your actions doesn't mean you should act as a doormat for other people's hostility. Remove yourself from people who hurt you, consistently don't trust you, or don't give you a fair shake.

Day 13

Far away there in the sunshine are my highest aspirations. I may not reach them, but I can look up and see their beauty, believe in them, and try to follow where they lead.

—*Louisa May Alcott*

Progressive Muscle Relaxation

Complete two 20-minute relaxation sessions—one with progressive muscle relaxation script 1 and one with progressive muscle relaxation script 2:

Yes, I completed session 1: ____
Yes, I completed session 2: ____

Before and after each session, rate your tension level on a scale from 1 to 10:

Session 1: My tension level before relaxation: ____
Session 1: My tension level after relaxation: ____
Session 2: My tension level before relaxation: ____
Session 2: My tension level after relaxation: ____

COGNITIVE BEHAVIOR THERAPY

Whenever you notice yourself in a bad mood, try to catch the thoughts that run through your head:

My mood: ＿＿＿
My mood's intensity (1 to 10): ＿＿＿
The situation:

My thoughts just before the mood set in:

TODAY'S TIP

Learn how to listen without interrupting others. Your interruptions make others perceive you as thinking that your ideas are more important than theirs. Holding your tongue may feel tough in the beginning, but it will get easier over time. Try making a game out of it: time yourself to see how long you can listen without talking. Once your friend, coworker, child, or spouse has finished talking, summarize what he or she has said. Then launch into what you want to say.

Day 14
I shall shape my future.
Whether I fail or succeed shall be no man's doing but my own.
I am the force; I can clear any obstacle before me.
Or I can be lost in the maze.
My choice. My responsibility.
Win or lose, only I hold the key to my destiny.

—Anonymous

Progressive Muscle Relaxation

Complete two 20-minute relaxation sessions—one with pro-gressive muscle relaxation script 1 and one with progressive muscle relaxation script 2:

    Yes, I completed session 1: _____
    Yes, I completed session 2: _____

Before and after each session, rate your tension level on a scale from 1 to 10:

    Session 1: My tension level before relaxation: _____
    Session 1: My tension level after relaxation: _____
    Session 2: My tension level before relaxation: _____
    Session 2: My tension level after relaxation: _____

Cognitive Behavior Therapy

Whenever you notice yourself in a bad mood, try to catch the thoughts that run through your head:

    My mood: _____
    My mood's intensity (1 to 10): _____
    The situation:

    My thoughts just before the mood set in:

Look back over your planner entries from week 2. Do you

notice a pattern to your thoughts, moods, and situations? If so, describe it here:

TODAY'S TIP

Get a pet. Research shows that people who care for a pet tend to feel calmer and experience better health than those who do not care for a pet. Perhaps the pet's continuous and unconditional love works to help us feel better. If you worry about your commitment and ability to care for an animal, start small with a goldfish rather than a dog. Once you know you can feed a fish every day, move on to a pet that requires more care.

Week 3

Put duties aside at least an hour before bed and perform soothing, quiet activities that will help you relax.

—*Dianne Hales, author*

During progressive muscle relaxation this week, you will begin your mini-relaxation sessions. Reread "Mini-Practices 101" in Chapter 7. The more you practice these sessions, the better you'll get at progressive muscle relaxation. Keep tabs on your tension levels throughout the day. Whenever you catch your heart racing, your palms sweating, or your muscles feeling tense, perform a short 30-second relaxation session, focusing on releasing the tension from all of the muscles in your body. If after 30 seconds you still don't feel relaxed, that's okay. Return to what you were doing, and try again later. For your formal sessions, you will continue to practice just once a day for 20 minutes, using script 2.

For cognitive behavior therapy this week, you will focus on testing the thoughts that you uncovered last week. Reread pages 110 to 112 in Chapter 8 to familiarize yourself with the topic, and make sure you have completed all of the suggested exercises in that section.

Day 15

Heroes are made in the hour of defeat. Success is, therefore,
well described as a series of glorious defeats.

—*Mohandas K. Gandhi*

PROGRESSIVE MUSCLE RELAXATION

Complete one 20-minute session with progressive muscle relaxation script 2, and start mini-practices as described in Chapter 7:

Yes, I completed session 1:____
Session 1: My tension level before relaxation (1 to 10): ____
Session 1: My tension level after relaxation (1 to 10): ____
I completed ____ mini-relaxation sessions today.

COGNITIVE BEHAVIOR THERAPY

Write down your moods and surrounding thoughts. Also, rate each thought for believability on a scale from 1 to 10. Analyze each thought by seeing if you've used flawed types of thinking (described on pages 110 to 111):

My mood: ____
The intensity of my mood (1 to 10): ____
The situation:

My thoughts:

How much I believe my thoughts (1 to 10): ____
These thoughts are examples of:

- All-or-nothing thinking   Y   N
- Overly general thinking   Y   N
- Mental filtering   Y   N
- Mental refereeing   Y   N
- Mind reading   Y   N
- Catastrophizing   Y   N
- Emotional thinking   Y   N
- "Should" thinking   Y   N
- Labeling   Y   N

Ask yourself the following questions:

What evidence supports these thoughts?
What evidence does not support my thoughts?
Have I jumped to conclusions?
Am I shouldering too much blame?
If a good friend knew about these thoughts, what would she or he tell me?
Are there any things that I am ignoring that could discount these thoughts?
Is there another way to see this situation?
How much I now believe my thoughts (1 to 10): ____

TODAY'S TIP

Recognize that all people are not the same. You're not abnormal because you think differently than someone else does. The same goes for anyone who doesn't think as you do. We all have unique viewpoints, ideas, feelings, moods, and actions. Practice accepting others just as they are and not as you wish them to be. Know that other people can disagree with you and still love you.

Day 16

Success isn't something you chase. It's something you have to put forth the effort for constantly. Then maybe it'll come when you least expect it. Most people don't understand that.

—*Michael Jordan*

PROGRESSIVE MUSCLE RELAXATION

Complete one 20-minute relaxation session with progressive muscle relaxation script 2. Continue doing mini-relaxation sessions for up to 30 seconds at a time whenever you feel tense:

Yes, I completed session 1: ____
Session 1: My tension level before relaxation (1 to 10): ____
Session 1: My tension level after relaxation (1 to 10): ____
I completed ____ mini-relaxation sessions today.

COGNITIVE BEHAVIOR THERAPY

Write down your moods and surrounding thoughts. Also, rate each thought for believability on a scale from 1 to 10. Analyze the thought by seeing if you've used flawed types of thinking (described on pages 110 to 111):

My mood: ____
The intensity of my mood (1 to 10): ____
The situation:

My thoughts:

How much I believe my thoughts (1 to 10): ____
These thoughts are examples of:

• All-or-nothing thinking   Y   N
• Overly general thinking   Y   N
• Mental filtering   Y   N

- Mental refereeing   Y   N
- Mind reading   Y   N
- Catastrophizing   Y   N
- Emotional thinking   Y   N
- "Should" thinking   Y   N
- Labeling   Y   N

What evidence supports these thoughts?

What evidence does not support my thoughts?

Have I jumped to conclusions?

Am I shouldering too much blame?

If a good friend knew about these thoughts, what would she or he tell me?

Are there any things that I am ignoring that could discount these thoughts?

Is there another way to see this situation?

How much I now believe my thoughts (1 to 10): ____

TODAY'S TIP

Sometimes the best way to handle your anger is to focus on something else until your mood and reactions subside. When you find your anger rising, find something to do: take a walk, immerse yourself in work, leaf through a magazine, divert yourself in some way, and, if you can, leave the immediate situation. If you can't leave the situation in the room, tell the person you are with that you have to stop discussing the topic until you can do so calmly.

Day 17

What lies behind us and what lies before us are tiny matters compared to what lies within us.

—*Ralph Waldo Emerson*

PROGRESSIVE MUSCLE RELAXATION

Complete one 20-minute relaxation session with progressive muscle relaxation script 2. Continue doing mini-relaxation sessions for up to 30 seconds at a time whenever you feel tense:

Yes, I completed session 1: ____
Session 1: My tension level before relaxation (1 to 10): ____
Session 1: My tension level after relaxation (1 to 10): ____
I completed ____ mini-relaxation sessions today.

COGNITIVE BEHAVIOR THERAPY

Write down your moods and surrounding thoughts. Also, rate each thought for believability on a scale from 1 to 10. Analyze the thought by seeing if you've used flawed types of thinking (described on pages 110 to 111):

My mood: ____
The intensity of my mood (1 to 10): ____
The situation:

My thoughts:

How much I believe my thoughts (1 to 10): ____
These thoughts are examples of:

• All-or-nothing thinking   Y   N
• Overly general thinking   Y   N
• Mental filtering   Y   N
• Mental refereeing   Y   N
• Mind reading   Y   N
• Catastrophizing   Y   N
• Emotional thinking   Y   N

- "Should" thinking   Y   N
- Labeling   Y   N

What evidence supports these thoughts?

What evidence does not support my thoughts?

Have I jumped to conclusions?

Am I shouldering too much blame?

If a good friend knew about these thoughts, what would she or he tell me?

Are there any things that I am ignoring that could discount these thoughts?

Is there another way to see this situation?

How much I now believe my thoughts (1 to 10): _____

TODAY'S TIP

There is great power in forgiveness, yet it's one of the hardest things to do. Rather than blame those who have treated you badly, forgive them. Let go of your resentment and anger and move on. You will often learn that your anger and resentment hurt you much more than the person you directed it toward. Forgiveness is really a gift to yourself rather than a gift for the other person.

Day 18

If you can DREAM it, you can DO it.

—*Walt Disney*

PROGRESSIVE MUSCLE RELAXATION

Complete one 20-minute relaxation session with progressive muscle relaxation script 2. Continue doing mini-relaxation sessions for up to 30 seconds at a time whenever you feel tense:

Yes, I completed session 1: _____

Session 1: My tension level before relaxation (1 to 10): _____

Session 1: My tension level after relaxation (1 to 10): _____

I completed _____ mini-relaxation sessions today.

Cognitive Behavior Therapy

Write down your moods and surrounding thoughts. Also, rate each thought for believability on a scale from 1 to 10. Analyze the thought by seeing if you've used flawed types of thinking (described on pages 110 to 111):

My mood: ____
The intensity of my mood (1 to 10): ____
The situation:

My thoughts:

How much I believe my thoughts (1 to 10): ____
These thoughts are examples of:

- All-or-nothing thinking   Y   N
- Overly general thinking   Y   N
- Mental filtering   Y   N
- Mental refereeing   Y   N
- Mind reading   Y   N
- Catastrophizing   Y   N
- Emotional thinking   Y   N
- "Should" thinking   Y   N
- Labeling   Y   N

What evidence supports these thoughts?
What evidence does not support my thoughts?
Have I jumped to conclusions?

Am I shouldering too much blame?

If a good friend knew about these thoughts, what would she or he tell me?

Are there any things that I am ignoring that could discount these thoughts?

Is there another way to see this situation?

How much I now believe my thoughts (1 to 10): _____

TODAY'S TIP

Whenever you feel unsure about how to handle a situation, check in with a friend or loved one who can be impartial. If you are not sure if your interpretation is accurate, ask a trusted friend about it and whether she or he would have responded the same way.

Day 19

When one door closes another door opens; but we so often look so long and so regretfully upon the closed door, that we do not see the ones which open for us.

—*Alexander Graham Bell*

PROGRESSIVE MUSCLE RELAXATION

Complete one 20-minute relaxation session with progressive muscle relaxation script 2. Continue doing mini-relaxation sessions for up to 30 seconds at a time whenever you feel tense:

Yes, I completed session 1: _____
Session 1: My tension level before relaxation (1 to 10): _____
Session 1: My tension level after relaxation (1 to 10): _____
I completed _____ mini-relaxation sessions today.

COGNITIVE BEHAVIOR THERAPY

Write down your moods and surrounding thoughts. Also, rate each thought for believability on a scale from 1 to 10. Analyze the thought by seeing if you've used flawed types of thinking (described on pages 110 to 111).

My mood: _____

The intensity of my mood (1 to 10): ____
The situation:

My thoughts:

How much I believe my thoughts (1 to 10): ____
These thoughts are examples of:

- All-or-nothing thinking   Y   N
- Overly general thinking   Y   N
- Mental filtering   Y   N
- Mental refereeing   Y   N
- Mind reading   Y   N
- Catastrophizing   Y   N
- Emotional thinking   Y   N
- "Should" thinking   Y   N
- Labeling   Y   N

What evidence supports these thoughts?
What evidence does not support my thoughts?
Have I jumped to conclusions?
Am I shouldering too much blame?
If a good friend knew about these thoughts, what would she or he tell me?
Are there any things that I am ignoring that could discount these thoughts?
Is there another way to see this situation?
How much I now believe my thoughts (1 to 10): ____

TODAY'S TIP

If you are shy, challenge yourself to talk to others. Say something nice to the cashier at the grocery store. Make comments to others waiting at the doctor's office. Make a point of saying hello to the mail carrier. The more connections you make, the more support you'll find, and the easier it will become for you to open up.

Day 20

Everything's in the mind. That's where it all starts. Knowing what you want is the first step toward getting it!

—*Mae West*

PROGRESSIVE MUSCLE RELAXATION

Complete one 20-minute relaxation session with progressive muscle relaxation script 2. Continue doing mini-relaxation sessions for up to 30 seconds at a time whenever you feel tense:

Yes, I completed session 1:____
Session 1: My tension level before relaxation (1 to 10): ____
Session 1: My tension level after relaxation (1 to 10): ____
I completed ____ mini-relaxation sessions today.

COGNITIVE BEHAVIOR THERAPY

Write down your moods and surrounding thoughts. Also, rate each thought for believability on a scale from 1 to 10. Analyze the thought by seeing if you've used flawed types of thinking (described on pages 110 to 111):

My mood: ____
The intensity of my mood (1 to 10): ____
The situation:

My thoughts:

How much I believe my thoughts (1 to 10): ____
These thoughts are examples of:

• All-or-nothing thinking   Y   N
• Overly general thinking   Y   N
• Mental filtering   Y   N
• Mental refereeing   Y   N
• Mind reading   Y   N
• Catastrophizing   Y   N
• Emotional thinking   Y   N
• "Should" thinking   Y   N
• Labeling   Y   N

What evidence supports these thoughts?
What evidence does not support my thoughts?
Have I jumped to conclusions?
Am I shouldering too much blame?
If a good friend knew about these thoughts, what would she or he tell me?
Are there any things that I am ignoring that could discount these thoughts?
Is there another way to see this situation?
How much I now believe my thoughts (1 to 10): ____

TODAY'S TIP

Compliment others, and watch how your words brighten their day. Make sure to say something that you really mean. Don't get frustrated if someone doesn't look happy after you've complimented him or her. Think back to your own ways of dealing with compliments in the past. Have you ever disregarded a compliment? Sometimes people feel embarrassed by attention or appreciation or are simply befuddled. They may be struggling with their own moods and problems.

Day 21

Everyone has inside him a piece of good news. The good news is that you don't yet realize how great you can be! How much you can accomplish! And what your potential is!

—*Anne Frank*

PROGRESSIVE MUSCLE RELAXATION

Complete one 20-minute relaxation session with script 2. Continue your mini-relaxation sessions for up to 30 seconds at a time whenever you feel tense:

Yes, I completed session 1: _____
Session 1: My tension level before relaxation (1 to 10): _____
Session 1: My tension level after relaxation (1 to 10): _____
I completed _____ mini-relaxation sessions today.

COGNITIVE BEHAVIOR THERAPY

Write down your moods and surrounding thoughts. Also, rate each thought for believability on a scale from 1 to 10. Analyze the thought by seeing if you've used flawed types of thinking (described on pages 110 to 111).

My mood: _____
The intensity of my mood (1 to 10): _____
The situation:

My thoughts:

How much I believe my thoughts (1 to 10): _____
These thoughts are examples of:

• All-or-nothing thinking   Y   N
• Overly general thinking   Y   N
• Mental filtering   Y   N
• Mental refereeing   Y   N
• Mind reading   Y   N
• Catastrophizing   Y   N
• Emotional thinking   Y   N
• "Should" thinking   Y   N
• Labeling   Y   N

What evidence supports these thoughts?
What evidence does not support my thoughts?
Have I jumped to conclusions?
Am I shouldering too much blame?
If a good friend knew about these thoughts, what would she or he tell me?
Are there any things that I am ignoring that could discount these thoughts?
Is there another way to see this situation?
How much I now believe my thoughts (1 to 10): _____

Look back over your planner entries from week 3. Do you notice a pattern or can you learn from your entries?

TODAY'S TIP

Receive compliments graciously. When someone says something nice to you, say, "Thank you." Don't try to explain away their positive information with comments such as, "Oh, that's not true." That response would hurt the feelings of the person giving the compliment. Also, write the compliment down in your journal at the end of the day. These compliments will become your evidence of the goodness in others and yourself when you are struggling with negativity.

Week 4

He enjoys true leisure who has time to improve his soul's estate.

—*Henry David Thoreau*

For progressive muscle relaxation this week, you will again focus on practicing relaxation in numerous mini-sessions throughout each day. Check off your mini-sessions as you complete them. The more often you practice, the better you will get. Aim for 10 to 20 mini-sessions a day. You may also do a formal relaxation session if you'd like, but it's not mandatory.

For cognitive behavior therapy this week, you will focus on uncovering the beliefs that lead to your negative thoughts. Reread pages 112 to 115 in Chapter 8 to familiarize yourself with this material and complete all of the suggested exercises.

Day 22

To love oneself is the beginning of a lifelong romance.

—*Oscar Wilde*

PROGRESSIVE MUSCLE RELAXATION

Try to complete between 10 and 20 mini-relaxation sessions:

Yes, I completed _____ mini-practice sessions.

COGNITIVE BEHAVIOR THERAPY

My mood: _____
Intensity of my mood (1 to 10): _____
Situation:

My thoughts:

Believability of my thoughts (1 to 10): ____
What these thoughts say about me: ____
What belief led to these thoughts: ____
Evidence that supports this belief:

Evidence that does not support this belief:

TODAY'S TIP

We all make mistakes, none of us is perfect. No matter how much you rethink a situation, you will eventually encounter one where you were wrong. The key here is to learn from it and move on rather than feel anxious, depressed, or angry about it. Whether you violate your own standards or those of someone else, say your apologies, make amends, and move on.

Day 23

Never tell your mom her diet's not working.
                    —*Michael, age 14, on various websites*

PROGRESSIVE MUSCLE RELAXATION

Try to complete between 10 and 20 mini-relaxation sessions:

Yes, I completed _____ mini-practice sessions.

COGNITIVE BEHAVIOR THERAPY

Write down your moods, the surrounding situation, and your thoughts. Rate each thought and look for evidence that supports or refutes its validity.

My mood: _____
Intensity of my mood (1 to 10): _____
The situation:

My thoughts:

Believability of my thoughts (1 to 10): _____
What these thoughts say about me: _____
What belief led to these thoughts: _____
Evidence that supports this belief:

Evidence that does not support this belief:

TODAY'S TIP

Schedule pleasurable activities into your life, especially if you scored high for depression in Chapter 6. Maximize the time you spend with others, and take part in activities that you enjoy. Think of five to ten activities right now, write them down, and make plans to engage in them this week. They might include meeting a friend for lunch, going for a walk in a park, listening to your favorite music, playing with your dog, or reading a book.

Day 24

Don't judge each day by the harvest you reap, but by the seeds you plant.

—*Robert Louis Stevenson*

PROGRESSIVE MUSCLE RELAXATION

Try to complete between ten and twenty mini-relaxation sessions:

Yes, I completed ____ mini-practice sessions.

COGNITIVE BEHAVIOR THERAPY

Write down your moods, the surrounding situation, and your thoughts. Rate each thought and look for evidence that supports or refutes its validity.

My mood: ____
Intensity of my mood (1 to 10): ____
The situation:

My thoughts:

Believability of my thoughts (1 to 10): ____
What these thoughts say about me: ____
What belief led to these thoughts: ____
Evidence that supports this belief:

Evidence that does not support this belief:

TODAY'S TIP
Reveal a secret to someone you trust. Holding in secrets takes a lot of mental energy and tends to make us feel unnecessarily guilty or ashamed. Do you have secrets that you keep from others? Do others know that you have diabetes? If not, start there. Then you can reveal your depression, anxiety, or hostility. Once you let your spouse or close friend know that you have recog-

nized an emotional problem and are taking steps to address and correct it, ask for his or her support.

Day 25
Keep away from people who try to belittle your ambitions.
Small people always do that, but the really great ones make
you feel that you, too, can become great.
                                              —*Mark Twain*

PROGRESSIVE MUSCLE RELAXATION

Try to complete between ten and twenty mini-relaxation sessions:

Yes, I completed __ mini-practice sessions.

COGNITIVE BEHAVIOR THERAPY

Write down your moods, the surrounding situation, and your thoughts. Rate each thought and look for evidence that supports or refutes its validity.

My mood: ____
Intensity of my mood (1 to 10): ____
The situation:

My thoughts:

Believability of my thoughts (1 to 10): ____

What these thoughts say about me: ____
What belief led to these thoughts: ____
Evidence that supports this belief:

Evidence that does not support this belief:

TODAY'S TIP

Use "I" statements whenever possible, particularly when talking about your feelings. If you need to ask someone why he or she has not been in touch, but say, "You didn't call me when I was sick to see if I needed help," you may put that person on the defensive. In contrast, stating, "I felt hurt and lonely when I didn't hear from you," allows for an emotional response and conversation. Although you may feel insecure talking about your feelings, you will find that you are more likely to get what you want when you speak in "I" statements.

Day 26

I like living. I have sometimes been wildly, despairingly, acutely miserable, racked with sorrow, but through it all I still know quite certainly that just to be alive is a great thing.
—*Agatha Christie*

PROGRESSIVE MUSCLE RELAXATION

Try to complete between ten and twenty mini-relaxation sessions:

Yes, I completed _____ mini-practice sessions.

COGNITIVE BEHAVIOR THERAPY

Write down your moods, the surrounding situation, and your thoughts. Rate each thought and look for evidence that supports or refutes its validity.

My mood: _____
Intensity of my mood (1 to 10): _____
The situation:

My thoughts:

Believability of my thoughts (1 to 10): _____
What these thoughts say about me: _____
What belief led to these thoughts: _____
Evidence that supports this belief:

Evidence that does not support this belief:

Today's Tip

Be your own devil's advocate. As you practice cognitive behavior therapy, it begins to become as automatic as progressive muscle relaxation. Give yourself mini-cognitive behavior therapy sessions. Continue to write down your formal sessions detailing situations, moods, and thoughts in your daily planner, but also try to do this process in your head as you notice thoughts or feelings. Reason with yourself, ask yourself if the mood or thought is valid, and consider whether there is another way to see the situation.

Day 27

You've got to think about "big things" while you're doing small things, so that all the small things go in the right direction.

—Alvin Toffler, futurist and writer

Progressive Muscle Relaxation

Try to complete between ten and twenty mini-relaxation sessions:

Yes, I completed _____ mini-practice sessions.

Cognitive Behavior Therapy

Write down your moods, the surrounding situation, and your thoughts. Rate each thought and look for evidence that supports or refutes its validity.

My mood: _____
Intensity of my mood (1 to 10): _____
The situation:

My thoughts:

Believability of my thoughts (1 to 10): _____
What these thoughts say about me: _____
What belief led to these thoughts: _____
Evidence that supports this belief: _____

Evidence that does not support this belief:

TODAY'S TIP
Learn how to speak up for your needs calmly. Sometimes we lash out at others because we anticipate a negative outcome. When letting someone know he or she hurt or disappointed you, focus on the behavior, not on the person. Say that the behavior is what you object to or that it distresses you, and say how the behavior makes you feel. Then say how you wish the person would treat you or behave in the future in similar situations.

Day 28

The difference between great people and everyone else is that great people create their lives actively, while everyone else is created by their lives, passively waiting to see where life takes them next. The difference between the two is the difference between living fully and just existing.
                    —Michael Gerber, business consultant and author

PROGRESSIVE MUSCLE RELAXATION

Try to complete between ten and twenty mini-relaxation sessions:

Yes, I completed _____ mini-practice sessions.

COGNITIVE BEHAVIOR THERAPY

Write down your moods, the surrounding situation, and your thoughts. Rate each thought and look for evidence that supports or refutes its validity.

My mood: _____
Intensity of my mood (1 to 10): _____
The situation:

My thoughts:

Believability of my thoughts (1 to 10): _____
What these thoughts say about me: _____

What belief led to these thoughts: _____
Evidence that supports this belief:

Evidence that does not support this belief:

TODAY'S TIP

Progressive muscle relaxation can help you overcome obsessive, hostile, or depressed thoughts. When you find yourself obsessing over something and can't seem to stop yourself, try a mini-practice session with this added technique: stare at a point in space and focus on relaxation for 30 seconds. This will help distract you from your thoughts. After 30 seconds, you may not be able to remember what you were obsessing about in the first place.

Look over your entries from the past week. Do you notice any patterns to your thinking?

Week 5

> *It's not stress that kills us, it is our reaction to it.*
>
> —*Hans Selye, physician*

For progressive muscle relaxation this week, you will continue with mini-practice sessions, using 30-second sessions to your advantage in more stressful situations.

For cognitive behavior therapy, you will examine old beliefs that you've gathered in your notes from last week. Each day you will examine one belief, and next to that belief write at least one alternate belief or assumption. Rate its believability on a scale from 1 to 10, with 1 being "very hard to believe" and 10 being "completely believable." Then you will gather evidence to test your alternate belief for accuracy.

Day 29

Just remember, 100% of the shots you don't take, don't go in.
—Wayne Gretzky

PROGRESSIVE MUSCLE RELAXATION

You may do a formal optional relaxation session if you'd like. However, focus on your mini-practices, trying to complete one whenever you notice you are tense. Complete between 10 and 20 mini-relaxation sessions.

Note your tension level before and after a few of your mini-sessions, rating it on a scale of 1 to 10:

My tension level before relaxation: _____
My tension level after relaxation: _____
My tension level before relaxation: _____
My tension level after relaxation: _____
My tension level before relaxation: _____
My tension level after relaxation: _____

COGNITIVE BEHAVIOR THERAPY

Write down your moods, the surrounding situation, and your thoughts and beliefs. List alternative beliefs and test them for accuracy.

My mood: _____
Intensity of my mood (1 to 10): _____
The situation:

The thoughts that led to the mood:

The belief that led to these thoughts:

Belief to be challenged:

How much I believe this (1 to 10): ____
Possible other beliefs that could also be true:

How much I believe this (1 to 10): ____
How I will test this new belief:

The outcome of my test:

What I've learned:

TODAY'S TIP

Changing your moods, thoughts, beliefs, and behaviors takes practice. If you begin to feel frustrated with the process, focus on the reasons you tackled this program. Not only will altering your beliefs help create a better, more relaxed, more enriched life, it will also help control your blood sugar and help reduce dangerous complications, thus allowing you to live longer. Make a list of why you want to change your thoughts, moods, and beliefs. Besides your health, they might include becoming a better spouse, friend, parent, or coworker.

Day 30

The thing always happens that you really believe in; and the belief in a thing makes it happen.

—*Frank Lloyd Wright*

PROGRESSIVE MUSCLE RELAXATION

You may do a formal optional relaxation session if you'd like. However, focus on your mini-practices, trying to complete one whenever you notice you are tense. Complete between 10 and 20 mini-relaxation sessions.

Note your tension level before and after a few of your mini-sessions, rating it on a scale of 1 to 10:

My tension level before relaxation: ____
My tension level after relaxation: ____
My tension level before relaxation: ____
My tension level after relaxation: ____
My tension level before relaxation: ____
My tension level after relaxation: ____

COGNITIVE BEHAVIOR THERAPY

Write down your moods, the surrounding situation, and your thoughts and beliefs. List alternative beliefs and test them for accuracy.

My mood: ____
Intensity of my mood (1 to 10): ____
The situation:

The thoughts that led to the mood:

The belief that led to these thoughts:

Belief to be challenged:

How much I believe this (1 to 10): ____
Possible other beliefs that could also be true:

How much I believe this (1 to 10): ____
How I will test this new belief:

The outcome of my test:

TODAY'S TIP
Notice your negative thoughts and view them as if you were a casual observer who can see which are valid and which are not. Negative, invalid thoughts will continue to pop up in your mind, but now when you notice a negative thought, you can turn it off. Your planner has taught you some patterns to your thinking. When you catch yourself thinking, "I'm not good enough" or "He's such an idiot," just say, "Stop it!" until the thought passes.

Day 31

Try not to become a man of success, but rather a man of value.

　　　　　　　　　　　　　　　　　　—*Albert Einstein*

PROGRESSIVE MUSCLE RELAXATION

You may do a formal optional relaxation session if you'd like. However, focus on your mini-practices, trying to complete one whenever you notice you are tense. Complete between 10 and 20 mini-sessions.

Note your tension level before and after a few of your mini-sessions, rating it on a scale of 1 to 10:

　　My tension level before relaxation: ＿＿＿
　　My tension level after relaxation: ＿＿＿
　　My tension level before relaxation: ＿＿＿
　　My tension level after relaxation: ＿＿＿
　　My tension level before relaxation: ＿＿＿
　　My tension level after relaxation: ＿＿＿

COGNITIVE BEHAVIOR THERAPY

Write down your moods, the surrounding situation, and your thoughts and beliefs. List alternative beliefs and test them for accuracy.

　　My mood: ＿＿＿
　　Intensity of my mood (1 to 10): ＿＿＿
　　The situation:

　　The thoughts that led to the mood:

The belief that led to these thoughts:

Belief to be challenged:

How much I believe this (1 to 10): _____
Possible other beliefs that could also be true:

How much I believe this (1 to 10): _____
How I will test this new belief:

The outcome of my test:

TODAY'S TIP

You've probably heard the phrase, "Put yourself in his shoes." When people irritate you or sadden you, try to look at things from their perspective. What might have caused them to say what they said?

Day 32

What happens is not as important as how you react to what happens.

—*Thaddeus Golas, author*

PROGRESSIVE MUSCLE RELAXATION

You may do a formal optional relaxation session if you'd like. However, focus on your mini-practices, trying to complete one whenever you notice you are tense. Complete between 10 and 20 mini-sessions.

Note your tension level before and after a few of your mini-sessions, rating it on a scale of 1 to 10:

My tension level before relaxation: ____
My tension level after relaxation: ____
My tension level before relaxation: ____
My tension level after relaxation: ____
My tension level before relaxation: ____
My tension level after relaxation: ____

COGNITIVE BEHAVIOR THERAPY

Write down your moods, the surrounding situation, and your thoughts and beliefs. List alternative beliefs and test them for accuracy.

My mood: ____
Intensity of my mood (1 to 10): ____
The situation:

The thoughts that led to the mood:

The belief that led to these thoughts:

Belief to be challenged:

How much I believe this (1 to 10): ____
Possible other beliefs that could also be true:

How much I believe this (1 to 10):____
How I will test this new belief:

The outcome of my test:

TODAY'S TIP

Do you routinely overextend yourself and then feel tired or burned out? Do you put the needs of others before your own? Do you put yourself last? Saying no can be hard. You may worry about disappointing someone, or you may think that if you say no, you're not as competent as you want to be. Saying yes too often, however, whittles away at your energy until you are no good to anyone. Take care of yourself first.

To gather the confidence to turn someone down, restate exactly what was asked of you: "You want me to [fill in the blank]." Then follow up with, "I know how important this is to you." Then say something like, "I'm sorry. I'd like to help, but I can't do that."

Day 33

No one can make you feel inferior without your consent.
                                                    —*Eleanor Roosevelt*

PROGRESSIVE MUSCLE RELAXATION

You may do a formal optional relaxation session if you'd like. However, focus on your mini-practices, trying to complete one whenever you notice you are tense. Complete between 10 and 20 mini-relaxation sessions.

Note your tension level before and after a few of your mini-sessions, rating it on a scale of 1 to 10:

My tension level before relaxation: _____
My tension level after relaxation: _____
My tension level before relaxation: _____
My tension level after relaxation: _____
My tension level before relaxation: _____
My tension level after relaxation: _____

COGNITIVE BEHAVIOR THERAPY

Write down your moods, the surrounding situation, and your thoughts and beliefs. List alternative beliefs and test them for accuracy.

My mood: _____
Intensity of my mood (1 to 10): _____
The situation:

The thoughts that led to the mood:

The belief that led to these thoughts:

Belief to be challenged:

How much I believe this (1 to 10): ____
Possible other beliefs that could also be true:

How much I believe this (1 to 10): ____
How I will test this new belief:

The outcome of my test:

Today's Tip
Laughter can provide some of the best medicine for a bad
mood. That's why some people deal with the strain of hard

times by telling jokes, even at seemingly inappropriate moments. It's hard to stay sad or angry when you are laughing. To start some chuckles, you might laugh at your own cynical thoughts or some other aspect of your thoughts or behavior. Or, at the end of a hard day, you might treat yourself to a funny movie or a night at a comedy club.

Day 34

I haven't failed, I've found 10,000 ways that don't work.

—*Ben Franklin*

PROGRESSIVE MUSCLE RELAXATION

You may do a formal optional relaxation session if you'd like, but focus on your mini-practices, trying to complete one whenever you notice you are tense. Complete between 10 and 20 mini-sessions.

Note your tension level before and after a few of your mini-sessions, rating it on a scale of 1 to 10:

My tension level before relaxation: _____
My tension level after relaxation: _____
My tension level before relaxation: _____
My tension level after relaxation: _____
My tension level before relaxation: _____
My tension level after relaxation: _____

COGNITIVE BEHAVIOR THERAPY

Write down your moods, the surrounding situation, and your thoughts and beliefs. List alternative beliefs and test them for accuracy.

My mood: _____
Intensity of my mood (1 to 10): _____
The situation:

The thoughts that led to the mood:

The belief that led to these thoughts:

Belief to be challenged:

How much I believe this (1 to 10): _____
Possible other beliefs that could also be true:

How much I believe this (1 to 10): _____

How I will test this new belief:

The outcome of my test:

TODAY'S TIP
Try to create opportunities to build trust in other people. For example, you might ask your hair stylist what he or she thinks would be the best cut for you rather than telling him or her exactly what you want each time. Or you might allow an employee to figure out a project without your guidance. Perhaps you could give your teenager more responsibility. You might let someone else drive the car and resist telling him or her when to turn or stop or put on a flasher. Keep track of the outcomes of these situations. You'll find that more often than not, people will exceed your expectations and help fuel your more positive outlook on the world.

Day 35

Life is not a matter of having good cards, but of playing a poor hand well.

—Robert Louis Stevenson

PROGRESSIVE MUSCLE RELAXATION
You may do a formal optional relaxation session if you'd like.

However, focus on your mini-practices, trying to complete one whenever you notice you are tense. Complete between 10 and 20 mini-sessions.

Note your tension level before and after a few of your mini-sessions, rating it on a scale of 1 to 10:

My tension level before relaxation: _____
My tension level after relaxation: _____
My tension level before relaxation: _____
My tension level after relaxation: _____
My tension level before relaxation: _____
My tension level after relaxation: _____

COGNITIVE BEHAVIOR THERAPY

Write down your moods, the surrounding situation, and your thoughts and beliefs. List alternative beliefs and test them for accuracy.

My mood: _____
Intensity of my mood (1 to 10): _____
The situation:

The thoughts that led to the mood:

The belief that led to these thoughts:

Belief to be challenged:

How much I believe this (1 to 10): _____
Possible other beliefs that could also be true:

How much I believe this (1 to 10): _____
How I will test this new belief:

The outcome of my test:

Look over your entries for the past week. Do you notice a pattern to your beliefs?

TODAY'S TIP

To lower your stress or hostility level, take steps to lower the stress of your surroundings. You can start by lessening the background noise in your own environment. Research shows that noise is very stressful, even for people who don't notice the noise around them. Do you really need to have the television on while you are talking on the phone? Does your teenage son need to play his music that loudly? Can you find a constructive way to ask your coworkers to hold their spirited conversations somewhere other than near your office door?

Week 6

A man who suffers or stresses before it is necessary, suffers more than is necessary.

—*Seneca*

By now, your relaxation efforts should feel almost automatic. You may find yourself going into a relaxed frame of mind and body without having been aware that you prompted yourself to do so. For the last week of your program, continue to monitor your tension levels and how often you practice relaxation.

For cognitive behavior therapy, you're ready to tackle your reactions to problems, moods, and situations. Reread Week 6 on pages 116 to 117 in Chapter 8, and complete any suggested preliminary exercises.

Day 36

You're good enough, you're smart enough, and gosh darn it people like you.

—*Stuart Smalley, Saturday Night Live character*

PROGRESSIVE MUSCLE RELAXATION

You may do a formal optional relaxation session if you'd like. However, focus on your mini-practices, trying to complete one whenever you notice you are tense. Complete between 10 and 20 mini-sessions.

Note your tension level before and after a few of your mini-sessions, rating it on a scale of 1 to 10:

My tension level before relaxation: _____
My tension level after relaxation: _____
My tension level before relaxation: _____
My tension level after relaxation: _____
My tension level before relaxation: _____
My tension level after relaxation: _____

COGNITIVE BEHAVIOR THERAPY

Pick a behavior you'd like to change and think of some solutions that could help you behave differently in the future. Then put your plan into practice.

Reaction I wish to address:

How else I might react in the future when in a similar situation:

Possible roadblocks I might encounter:

How I will deal with those roadblocks:

TODAY'S TIP

When you know you may be facing a situation that will cause you stress or make you angry, you may be able to prepare for it and avoid emotional upheaval. Use relaxation techniques before the encounter to keep your mind and body calm. While relaxed, visualize the upcoming encounter. Where are you? What are you saying? Who are you with? Whenever you feel signs of stress, return to the relaxation exercise. Once you are calm, return to your visualization. See yourself speaking your mind calmly. See and hear problems arise during the conversation, and visualize yourself responding to them calmly but assertively.

When you encounter the actual situation, you will have prepared your body to stay calm and your mind to know what to say.

Day 37

I am always doing that which I can not do, in order that I may learn how to do it.

—*Pablo Picasso*

PROGRESSIVE MUSCLE RELAXATION

You may do a formal optional relaxation session if you'd like. However, focus on your mini-practices, trying to complete one whenever you notice you are tense. Complete between 10 and 20 mini-sessions.

Note your tension level before and after a few of your mini-sessions, rating it on a scale of 1 to 10:

My tension level before relaxation: _____
My tension level after relaxation: _____
My tension level before relaxation: _____
My tension level after relaxation: _____

My tension level before relaxation: ____
My tension level after relaxation: ____

COGNITIVE BEHAVIOR THERAPY

Pick a behavior you'd like to change and think of some solutions that could help you behave differently in the future. Then put your plan into practice.

Reaction I wish to address:

How else I might react in the future when in a similar situation:

Possible roadblocks I might encounter:

How I will deal with those roadblocks:

My outcome:

TODAY'S TIP

Scan your body regularly for signs of stress, anger, fear, or sadness. Try to notice shakiness, muscle tension, chest pressure, clenched or sweaty palms, and other signs at their earliest stage. Noticing negative emotions as they are beginning to emerge will help you better direct your behavior during the surrounding situation.

Day 38

A pessimist is one who makes difficulties of his opportunities, and an optimist is one who makes opportunities of his difficulties.

—*Harry Truman*

PROGRESSIVE MUSCLE RELAXATION

You may do a formal optional relaxation session if you'd like. However, focus on your mini-practices, trying to complete one whenever you notice you are tense. Complete between 10 and 20 mini-sessions.

Note your tension level before and after a few of your mini-sessions, rating it on a scale of 1 to 10:

My tension level before relaxation: _____
My tension level after relaxation: _____
My tension level before relaxation: _____
My tension level after relaxation: _____
My tension level before relaxation: _____
My tension level after relaxation: _____

COGNITIVE BEHAVIOR THERAPY

Pick a behavior you'd like to change and think of some solutions that could help you behave differently in the future. Then put your plan into practice.

Reaction I wish to address:

How else I might react in the future when in a similar situation:

Possible roadblocks I might encounter:

How I will deal with those roadblocks:

TODAY'S TIP

Take time-outs. When you feel angry, upset, or emotional,

remove yourself from the situation. Go outside for a walk, or
find a quiet place to be by yourself. This will give you time to
think over the situation, calm down, and arrive at an effective
solution. Regroup, relax, and restrategize. Allow your time-out
to last as long as needed, but don't use it as an escape. When
you're calm, confront your problem assertively.

Day 39

*A man who stands on a hill with his mouth open will wait a
long time for a roast duck to drop in.*

—Confucius

PROGRESSIVE MUSCLE RELAXATION

You may do a formal optional relaxation session if you'd like.
However, focus on your mini-practices, trying to complete one
whenever you notice you are tense. Complete between 10 and
20 mini-sessions.

Note your tension level before and after a few of your mini-
sessions, rating it on a scale of 1 to 10:

My tension level before relaxation: ____
My tension level after relaxation: ____
My tension level before relaxation: ____
My tension level after relaxation: ____
My tension level before relaxation: ____
My tension level after relaxation: ____

COGNITIVE BEHAVIOR THERAPY

Pick a behavior you'd like to change and think of some solutions
that could help you behave differently in the future. Then put
your plan into practice.

Reaction I wish to address:

How else I might react in the future when in a similar situation:

Possible roadblocks I might encounter:

How I will deal with those roadblocks:

TODAY'S TIP

The more assertive you are, the less people will take advantage of you. Practice asking for what you need, making requests of other people, and confronting situations. When you confront someone, remember to focus on that person's behavior and not on his or her personality in general. Avoid "always" statements; instead remain specific about the time, place, and other facts of the situation.

Day 40

Doing the best at this moment puts you in the best place for the next moment.

—*Oprah Winfrey*

PROGRESSIVE MUSCLE RELAXATION

You may do a formal optional relaxation session if you'd like. However, focus on your mini-practices, trying to complete one whenever you notice you are tense. Complete between 10 and 20 mini-sessions.

Note your tension level before and after a few of your mini-sessions, rating it on a scale of 1 to 10:

My tension level before relaxation: ____
My tension level after relaxation: ____
My tension level before relaxation: ____
My tension level after relaxation: ____
My tension level before relaxation: ____
My tension level after relaxation: ____

COGNITIVE BEHAVIOR THERAPY

Pick a behavior you'd like to change and think of some solutions that could help you behave differently in the future. Then put your plan into practice.

Reaction I wish to address:

How else I might react in the future when in a similar situation:

Possible roadblocks I might encounter:

How I will deal with those roadblocks:

TODAY'S TIP

You tell people more about your thoughts through your body language than through your words or actions. How you stand, your facial expression, even how quickly or in what tone you speak tells others if you are annoyed, happy, sad, or angry. When communicating with others, try to match your body language to your intent. If you are apologizing but do so through tight lips, you won't be taken seriously. If you worry that your body language will give you away, confront someone in writing rather than in person.

Day 41

Now is the only time there is. Make your now wow, your minutes miracles, and your days pay. Your life will have been magnificently lived and invested, and when you die you will have made a difference.

—*Mark Victor Hansen, motivational speaker and writer*

PROGRESSIVE MUSCLE RELAXATION

You may do a formal optional relaxation session if you'd like. However, focus on your mini-practices, trying to complete one whenever you notice you are tense. Complete between 10 and 20 mini-sessions.

Note your tension level before and after a few of your mini-sessions, rating it on a scale of 1 to 10:

My tension level before relaxation: _____
My tension level after relaxation: _____
My tension level before relaxation: _____
My tension level after relaxation: _____
My tension level before relaxation: _____
My tension level after relaxation: _____

COGNITIVE BEHAVIOR THERAPY

Pick a behavior you'd like to change and think of some solutions that could help you behave differently in the future. Then put your plan into practice.

Reaction I wish to address:

How else I might react in the future when in a similar situation:

Possible roadblocks I might encounter:

How I will deal with those roadblocks:

TODAY'S TIP

If you are shy and tend to avoid people, start practicing new behaviors by joining conversations. When you join a conversation, introduce yourself, if needed, and ask others about themselves. Most people enjoy talking about themselves. You'll be surprised how attracted people will be to you once you allow them to open up and become the center of your attention.

Day 42

In the midst of movement and chaos, keep stillness inside of you.

—*Deepak Chopra*

PROGRESSIVE MUSCLE RELAXATION

You may do a formal optional relaxation session if you'd like. However, focus on your mini-practices, trying to complete one whenever you notice you are tense. Complete between 10 and 20 mini-sessions.

Note your tension level before and after a few of your mini-sessions, rating it on a scale of 1 to 10:

My tension level before relaxation: _____
My tension level after relaxation: _____
My tension level before relaxation: _____
My tension level after relaxation: _____
My tension level before relaxation: _____
My tension level after relaxation: _____

Cognitive Behavior Therapy

Pick a behavior you'd like to change and think of some solutions that could help you behave differently in the future. Then put your plan into practice.

Reaction I wish to address:

How else I might react in the future when in a similar situation:

Possible roadblocks I might encounter:

How I will deal with those roadblocks:

Today's Tip

Weigh your options. If you're on the fence about whether to solve a problem, confront someone, or just let it go, ask yourself these questions: "Am I or someone I love truly being mistreated? Do I have effective options to change this situation? Is it worth the effort to get this person to change?" If your answer is yes to all three, use your assertiveness and problem-solving skills to address the problem.

CONGRATULATIONS

You've successfully completed the six-week program. I hope you are feeling more relaxed, that any depression has lifted, and that your angry moods have decreased in frequency. Keep in mind that this isn't the end of the program for you. It is actually just the beginning. You must continue to practice these techniques on a regular basis to keep stress and tension in check, your thoughts focused on the positive, and your reactions assertive.

It's like getting on the scale every day to control your weight. If you let a lot of time go by between weigh-ins, you may not notice a little indiscretion here and a little indulgence there, and the pounds may creep on before you know it. It's the same with relaxation and positive thinking. You must practice regularly in order to stay on an even keel.

You may have already experienced an improvement in blood sugar control, but it's possible that this improvement may take a little more time, as long as six months. Don't give up or think yourself a failure. Look back to your planner entries for proof that you've changed your outlook and improved your life.

If you find that your moods did not improve and that your blood sugar is the same or even worse after six months, turn to Chapters 11 and 13 for information on drugs that may help, as well as where to get professional help. If your physician has told you that you are overweight and that those extra pounds may be keeping you from controlling your blood sugar, turn to Chapter 10 for a mind-body program designed to help you lose weight.

Part III

Additional Things You Can Do: Drugs, Herbs, and Other Behavioral Approaches

10

Appetite Awareness

A Mind-Body Program for Eating Less and Losing Weight

WEIGHT control is a powerful way to lower blood sugar levels. Although obesity isn't a mental barrier to diabetes, it aggravates diabetes greatly. First and most important, it makes your body cells less sensitive to insulin. That means your body needs more insulin to shuttle blood sugar into cells, which means your pancreas overworks itself on a regular basis. When you lose weight and improve insulin sensitivity, you end up with a nice side effect that may help you along your weight-loss journey: lower insulin levels tend to lower hunger levels.

Some very new mind-body techniques have been developed recently to help you eat less and lose weight. These techniques are based on cognitive behavior therapy, which you learned about in Chapter 8, so they will feel familiar to you. I have not made these new techniques part of the six-week program because I did not want to overwhelm you with too many things to do at once. So if you have not yet begun working on the techniques reviewed up to this point, begin the program as outlined in Part II before attempting appetite awareness.

This mind-body appetite awareness program works because it does the exact opposite of many diets, which impose a strict set of rules, says psychologist Linda Craighead, a professor of psychology who developed many of these techniques Her program is revolutionary. Instead of restricting calories and certain foods, you will adopt a healthful eating approach that focuses on realistic portion sizes. This will help you reduce your weight, maintain better blood sugar control, normalize cholesterol levels, and prevent some of the complications of diabetes.

The mind-body techniques presented in this chapter do not force you to follow a specific diet with an outline of specific foods and amounts. Many physicians and nutritionists are beginning to shy away from stringent recommendations of calories and grams of carbohydrate, protein, and fat. (For more information on healthy eating, consult the resource list in Chapter 13.) Nutritionists and physicians now opt to take a look at what you are eating and how much you exercise, and then suggest strategic changes that you can live with and maintain for the rest of your life. In line with this approach, this chapter presents six simple life strategies to help you use your mind—and your body—to eat less, feel more satisfied, and lose weight. Use them every day, and you will lose weight and keep it off.

The Downfall of Dieting

In case you ever feel tempted to speed weight loss along by restricting your food intake and allowing yourself to become too hungry, post the following list and read it often:

Dieting . . .
• Makes you feel deprived.
• Eliminates the joys and pleasures of eating.
• Focuses on willpower rather than realism.
• Focuses your body, mind, and soul on food.
• Creates cravings.
• Reinforces the food mood cycle.
• Creates guilt, which can lead to overeating.

Test Your Overeating Behavior

To find out whether you need to work on appetite awareness, rate your hunger on a scale from 1 to 10 (with 1 being ravenous and 10 being stuffed) before and after each meal for a week. Keep track of your eating habits in your notebook by setting up the following worksheet:

DAY 1

Prebreakfast hunger level: ____

Postbreakfast hunger level: ____

Prelunch hunger level: ____

Postlunch hunger level: ____

Predinner hunger level: ____

Postdinner hunger level: ____

(Make similar notebook charts for Days 2 through 7.)

After one week, look over your ratings. If you rated your hunger an 8 or above more than seven times *after* a meal, you are a good candidate for the appetite awareness program. If you rated your hunger at a 1 or 2 seven or more times *before* a meal during the week, you are also a good candidate for this program. If you experienced difficulty rating your hunger at all, you also will benefit from this program. Finally, if your doctor has suggested that you need to lose weight, appetite awareness will help.

Remember to tackle the appetite awareness program *after* you have successfully mastered the skills described in Chapters 7 through 9.

Basic Information About Weight to Keep and Renew

Before learning appetite awareness, fill out the following. It will help you to see just how much progress you've made at the end of the six-week program:

My weight is: ____

According to the "Test Your Overeating Behavior" quiz, overeating is a problem for me. Y N

I tend to overeat (a) nearly every day, (b) most days, (c) once a week, (d) every once in a while, (e) rarely.

I eat because of stress or a negative emotion (a) nearly every day, (b) most days, (c) once a week, (d) every once in a while, (e) rarely.

WHY YOU OVEREAT

Obesity is a complex problem that is related to genetics and your living environment. Many people, myself included, have multiple thrifty genes that cause us to store energy very easily as fat. Genetics is not the only problem behind weight gain. Lifestyle also contributes to the problem. In addition to exercising less, we are eating more. There is so much food available that we have learned to ignore many of the natural cues that used to help us control our food intake. Food is often a source of recreation in our society. We eat for fun, not for nutrition.

Other factors may also cause you to reach for certain foods when you are not hungry. Some foods may have become intricately intertwined with memories. Just as you may avoid certain foods that you associate with negative memories (such as foods you ate just before coming down with the stomach flu), you may gravitate to foods that you associate with positive emotions, such as birthday cake for a party, mashed potatoes for comfort, or pizza for a celebration.

Your memories of good and bad times during childhood and how they relate to food may be in part why you turn to food during a crisis. Did your mother or father feed you certain foods to help lift your spirits when you were younger? If they did, you probably turn to those same foods today for the same reasons. Food has cultural, personal, and emotional power. In order to lose weight, you must take a good hard look at *why* you eat when you are really not hungry—that is, why you overeat. Once you know those answers, you will be able to use your mind to help control your eating.

BE REALISTIC ABOUT WEIGHT LOSS

Too often, we set our weight-loss goals too high and then get discouraged, which leads to backsliding and, in the end, weight gain. Aim for losing only 5 to 10 percent of your total weight. For example, if you weigh 220, a safe and healthy weight loss would be 11 to 22 pounds. Research shows that this is all you need to lose to result in better blood sugar control.

THE APPETITE AWARENESS PROGRAM

Now you're ready to start your appetite awareness program. I recommend you keep a notebook handy as you follow the program. Jot down thoughts, information, and ideas every day.

Week 1: Tune in to Your Appetite

Now you're ready to start your appetite awareness program. I recommend you keep a notebook handy as you follow the program. Jot down thoughts, information, and ideas every day. Your first step in the appetite awareness program involves tuning into your appetite. Many people are completely out of touch with their natural hunger signals. If you've dieted many times during your life, you may be one of them. When you diet and deprive yourself of food, you teach your body to tune out natural feelings of hunger: the rumble in your stomach, the sensation of an empty stomach, and the symptoms that stem from going too long without eating, such as headache and fatigue. Similarly, if you chronically binge or overeat, you're probably also out of touch with your hunger signals. When you eat well beyond your sensations of fullness, you lose touch with the subtle body cues that tell you when your stomach is getting too full.

One of the most important steps in using your mind to lose weight is getting back in touch with these natural hunger signals. Doing so will help prevent those crazed "I'm starving" kitchen raids. It will help stop you from overeating at Thanksgiving and other holiday feasts. You'll be able to navigate just about any eating situation without feeling tempted to overdo it.

True hunger has definite physical feelings: a rumbling, empty feeling in your stomach, perhaps a headache or light-headedness. You want to learn to eat before the headache and light-headedness set in. *When you are overhungry, you tend to overeat.*

In the appetite awareness training, you follow three simple rules.

1. *Eat long before you feel ravenous.* If you wait too long, you will make poor food choices, eat too quickly, and generally eat too much. To make sure you don't get too hungry, follow a regular schedule of planned meals and snacks. If you teach your body to expect food at certain times, it will adapt to the sched-

ule and will be less likely to give you false hunger signals. Some people feel comfortable eating the typical three meals a day, but Linda Craighead recommends three meals and two or three planned snacks. Find a pattern that works for you.

2. *Try to eat only when you feel physically hungry.* You will still eat your planned meals and snacks, but you will not begin to eat until you feel hungry. If you can do this, you will eliminate a lot of emotional and mindless eating. If you develop a craving for something, tell yourself you can have it, but wait until you feel hungry to eat it.

If you graze all day and never actually feel hungry, you may not be able to recognize when you feel satisfied. Craighead believes that we must allow ourselves to experience a sense of pleasure from eating. This pleasure helps you learn the difference between filling your stomach to a comfortable amount and overfilling it. Giving yourself permission to enjoy what you eat helps you realize that you do not need to overeat. Eventually, overeating won't feel as good as eating a normal amount.

3. *Stop eating before you feel stuffed.* Each time you eat beyond fullness, you grow more out of touch with your body's signals and don't feel satisfied with normal amounts of food. Some people try to get satisfied by eating very large amounts of low-calorie foods, but this strategy usually backfires. If you are used to large quantities of food, you will also tend to eat large quantities of high-calorie foods when they are available.

So how do you tune in to your hunger? As you've done in previous mind-body programs, use a rating scale from 1 to 10, with 1 equaling ravenous and 10 feeling stuffed. Begin to eat when you rate your hunger between a 3 or 4, and always try to eat before your hunger level dips below 3, before you become too hungry. Then stop eating once your fullness level reaches a 6 or 7 on your scale. Stopping once you reach 5 is too early. That's before the pleasure and satisfaction of eating kick in, says Craighead. You must allow yourself to feel satisfied on a daily basis. Aim to feel satisfied but not stuffed.

You will do this for several weeks. During the first week, you will start with just noticing your hunger. Once you are tuned in to your hunger, try to follow the rating scale, starting to eat at a level 3 or 4 and stopping at a 6 or 7. Keep notes about your successes and challenges. If you have a lot of difficulty tuning in to your hunger and fullness, Craighead says, you may be caught in one of the following five cycles:

- "EMOTIONAL EATING" CYCLE. This is when food becomes your main coping strategy to deal with stress, depression, anger, and other emotions and moods. The more you reinforce this pattern, the harder it is to break out of it. If you think you are caught in this cycle, revisit cognitive behavior therapy in Chapter 8. You will also find additional ways to deal with the emotional eating cycle in subsequent steps of this program.
- "FOOD AVAILABLE" CYCLE. You eat when you see food. Perhaps coworkers bring treats into the office. Or you pile up your plate at a buffet. Or you eat because someone else is eating and you don't want him or her to feel left out. We are genetically hardwired to eat when we see food, but because food is everywhere, you may need to take special steps to make sure the sights and smells of food don't trigger you to ignore your "I'm full" signals.
- "IGNORE HUNGER/TOO HUNGRY" CYCLE. This is the dieting cycle. You feel hungry but you refuse to give into those cues—until it's too late. Craighead particularly stresses that you should never "diet" because dieting is the opposite of appetite awareness. When you diet and deprive yourself of food, you force yourself to ignore your natural hunger and appetite, which causes you to become more and more out of touch with these natural urges. To help break this cycle, Craighead suggests that you eat three meals and two snacks a day. This will keep you out of the "ignore hunger" cycle. But don't become rigid about following a pattern. The goal here is to tune in to your hunger. "If you are following a schedule that works for you, you will usually be a little hungry when you decide to eat," she says.
- "IGNORE FULLNESS" CYCLE. This is the cycle that you get into when you overeat well beyond your feelings of fullness. We've all done this from time to time, most often at restaurants and holiday celebrations, when food is very readily available and

very tempting. "The best way to beat this cycle is to stay very aware, or some would say be very mindful, whenever you are eating," says Craighead. "You need to make all eating a conscious choice and to check in with yourself often while you are eating so you can stop just as soon as you feel comfortably satiated."

• "WHAT THE HECK" CYCLE. This results from the all-or-nothing thinking that I mentioned in Chapter 8. Once you break your "ignore hunger" cycle and eat a forbidden food or cheat in some way on your diet, you tend to have thoughts such as, "Now I've blown it. Why bother? I might as well eat as much as I want." This leads to further overeating.

Tuning in to your body's signals is the first step to recovering from overeating. Congratulate yourself for simply noticing how you feel when you start eating and when you stop. Don't berate yourself for going overboard. Guilt will only make problems worse. Congratulate yourself for tuning in and noticing whenever you eat beyond feelings of fullness. The more you tune in, the better you'll be able to stop eating before you overdo it.

Be patient with yourself. The more often you tune in to hunger and start eating only when you feel hungry and stop eating when you feel moderately full, the more natural the process will become. Don't worry if it feels hard at first. Eventually your body will readjust.

In Your Notebook

For week 1, use your notebook to help you keep track of your hunger and eating habits. Do not worry about how you respond to hunger at this point. Just notice when you feel hungry and when you feel full, particularly when you eat beyond feelings of fullness. Before and after each meal and snack, rate your hunger and fullness on the 1 to 10 scale. A sample day in your notebook might look like this:

Prebreakfast hunger level: 1
Postbreakfast hunger level: 9

Presnack hunger level: 1
Postsnack hunger level: 8
Prelunch hunger level: 4
Postlunch hunger level: 7
Presnack hunger level: 1
Postsnack hunger level: 9
Predinner hunger level: 3
Postdinner hunger level: 8

At the end of the week, look back over your notes. Do you notice a pattern to your pre- and postmeal hunger levels? If so, write down some thoughts, and then move on to the exercises for week 2.

Week 2: Get in Touch

In addition to monitoring your hunger signals, you must find out what causes you to overeat. To do so you'll look at the who, what, where, why, and how of your eating habits. In particular, you'll zero in on why. Examining why you eat may be the most important step to learning how to eat less and lose weight.

In Your Notebook

During each meal and snack, jot down what you ate, how much you ate, when you ate, and the situation surrounding your eating—just as you did in the cognitive behavior therapy chapter. Jot down who you were with, what you were doing just before you ate, and where you were—any and all details that may serve as clues to discovering why you overate. Also rate your hunger on a 1 to 10 scale before and after each meal, but also jot down notes that help describe why you eat the way you do. A sample entry in your notebook might look something like this:

Predinner hunger level: 1
Postdinner hunger level: 10

Comments: The situation surrounding the meal: I came home from work still feeling angry with my boss for piling on extra work at the last minute. I didn't get a chance to eat much for lunch or a snack either, so I was ravenous. As I made dinner, I nibbled on the ingredients and snacked on crackers. I couldn't stop thinking about my boss and a few comments he had made today. I kept thinking that I must not be good enough to do this job. I poured myself a glass of wine to help myself calm down. I felt terrible after dinner, almost sick.

Jot down the thoughts that ran through your mind just before eating as well as the mood you felt and its intensity just before eating. Do this every day for a week. At the end of the week, examine your journal for clues. You may find that you tend to overeat when you're with a particular person, when you're in a particular mood, or when you find yourself thinking about a particular memory.

After one week of journal keeping, you will have made important discoveries about your eating personality. Reflect about how well self-monitoring has worked for you. Are you now aware why you eat?

Many studies have shown that people who are willing to keep a food journal are more successful in losing weight than those who do not. Some people find self-monitoring very helpful and don't mind doing it. If self-monitoring works for you, keep it up for as long as you are trying to lose weight.

If you find self-monitoring too difficult to keep up all the time or you don't like doing it, keep track of only your most problematic times. For example, if you have little difficulty during the week, you may need to keep a food journal only during weekends. If you tend to gain weight over holidays or vacations, make a special effort to write in your food journal during those times. If your only problem is after-dinner snacking, just keep track of that.

The important thing is to understand that keeping a food diary is an important tool. Anytime you hit a plateau, feel as if you are getting off track, or don't understand why you are gaining weight, go back to self-monitoring. Many people find it very helpful to keep their food journal one week during each month. It keeps them honest and prevents slipping back into old habits.

Week 3: Address Your Stress-Eating Connection

Nearly all of us at one time or another have turned to food when we are under stress. Strong hunger signals after stress would have worked to help our ancestors survive physical threats, which involved burning calories while running away from wild animals or burning calories while fighting, such as clubbing a wild animal to death. These days we rarely burn calories in order to secure our survival. Indeed, we most often trigger the fight-or-flight response due to emotional stress rather than physical stress. We don't physically run away from a deadline at work; rather, we sit at our desk and peck frantically at a keyboard. Yet our bodies cannot distinguish well between mental and physical threats, and the brain responds to both by issuing a call for calories.

Some people eat when they experience stress because it provides an outlet or diversion—a way to procrastinate. For example, rather than completing that project on time, you go to the cafeteria and order coffee and bagel. Fortunately, the progressive muscle relaxation technique you learned in Chapter 7 will help you reduce such stressful episodes.

Here are some mind-body tips to help you break your stress-eating cycle:

• Refocus your attention on your mini-practice progressive muscle relaxation sessions, aiming for twenty mini-practices a day. When you are under stress and find yourself reaching for food, do a mini–progressive muscle relaxation session. Take about 20 seconds and focus on relaxing, mentally telling your muscles to let go.

• Look over your food diary. Are there any situations where you found yourself eating when under stress? Take a few moments to think about what else you could have done instead of turning to food. Could you have gone for a walk? How about talking with a coworker? Think of some noneating outlets for your stress. Devise a stress solution for every place you usually find yourself: home, work, and social settings. For example, choosing "taking a bath" as a way to relieve stress works great at home but not at work. You want a solution to turn to for every situation in which you find yourself.

• Never eat while doing something else, such as driving, reading, or working. Allowing yourself to focus fully on the task at hand—eating—will help keep you from stressing out. As your stress dissipates, so will your desire for food.

In Your Notebook

Monitor your hunger levels before and after each meal, aiming to start eating at a 3 or 4 on your scale and stop eating when your hunger reaches a 6 or 7 on the scale. In addition, each day jot down ways you can prevent stress from driving you to eat. Before each meal, perform a mini-relaxation session, using progressive muscle relaxation to help prevent stress-induced eating.

An entry in your notebook might look like this:

I completed my mini-relaxation session: Yes
Prelunch hunger level: 2
Postlunch hunger level: 6

Comments: Just before lunch, I got a call about my sick grandmother. I felt terrible about her health. Then I did my mini-relaxation session. Though I still felt bad, I didn't feel as frantic or stressed about her condition. I was able to eat more slowly as a result.

Step 4: Solve Your Problems

Once you know why you overeat, it is time to take control of the triggers that make you eat. First, know that *you* are in control. You cannot blame family and friends for your overeating or your boss for the stress that causes you to eat. You must be confident that you are ready to change. You can do something about your weight now and you will do something about it. As the old adage goes, "If you think you can, you will."

This week, you will think up possible solutions to help surmount the reasons that cause you to overeat or eat when you are not hungry. To help get the creative juices flowing, consult this list of possible solutions to common overeating problems.

COMMON OVEREATING TRIGGER: Stress
POSSIBLE SOLUTIONS: Progressive muscle relaxation session; going for a quick walk; calling a friend; asking someone to help you accomplish your to-do list
COMMON OVEREATING TRIGGER: Feeling the need to eat everything on your plate
POSSIBLE SOLUTIONS: Switching to a smaller dinner plate; asking for "half" restaurant portions; sharing your meal with a friend
COMMON OVEREATING TRIGGER: Craving certain foods to the point of dreaming about them
POSSIBLE SOLUTIONS: Eating snacks to make sure you don't get overhungry; allowing yourself small, controlled portions of your favorite foods every day
COMMON OVEREATING TRIGGER: Social events
POSSIBLE SOLUTIONS: Bringing the low-calorie healthy dish to parties; eating a small snack before you arrive to prevent feeling overhungry; staying away from the food table

In Your Notebook

Look at the clues that you uncovered about your eating habits in your eating journal. Besides stress, what else tends to make you overeat? List the people, moods, events, and situations that tend to trigger an overeating episode.

Once you know the clues, you can solve the problems that cause overeating. Think of overeating as a simple problem that you can solve with a little thought and trial and error. Rather than forcing yourself to "eat less" or "lose weight," you'll solve smaller, more doable problems such as "not bingeing on mashed potatoes" or "leaving a restaurant without feeling stuffed."

Next to each problem situation, mood, or person on your list, jot down three to four positive solutions to your problem. Perhaps you can meet a friend in a location that doesn't involve food. Maybe you can find ways to address the mood that causes you to eat.

Continue to monitor your hunger levels, aiming to begin eating at a 3 or 4 and stop by a 6 or 7 on your scale. For example, one entry in your journal might look like this:

Problem that causes me to overeat: My spouse makes negative comments about my appearance, making me feel terrible

Three ways I can address this problem: (1) Talk to my spouse about how these comments make me feel. (2) Vent to a friend about these comments. (3) Find a funny quip to shoot back, such as "There's more of me to love."

Week 5: Create a Support Team

Much research shows that you can more easily acquire a new habit—whether it's tuning in to your hunger or starting an exercise program—when you have a strong support team behind you. The support you receive from family and friends can help prevent you from emotionally beating yourself up and allowing guilt to fuel your eating. You can turn to family and friends rather than food during times of stress, sadness, frustration, or anger. To build your support team, let others know what you are trying to do. The more secretive you are about your efforts, the more easily you will give up. Choose friends and family whom you can call, visit, or e-mail when you need to. Just as you did in Chapter 8, you will now pick at least three members for your support team: a health supporter, a chore supporter, and an emotional supporter.

Your health supporter will help remind you of the many benefits of your recent changes and can help you chronicle your weight loss. Your chore supporter will help ease the burdens that prevent you from eating healthfully or from exercising. For example, if you don't have food available, it will be difficult to sit down to a meal whenever you feel hungry. Your chore supporter might offer to run to the grocery store to stock the kitchen.

You may need more than one emotional supporter. You never know when an emotion will drive you to the refrigerator, and you need a big support team so that you can get in touch with someone at that moment. If you commonly find yourself raiding the fridge in the middle of the night, you might try finding support on the Internet in a weight-loss chatroom. You might not want to wake up a friend in the middle of the night with a call, but you can log onto the Internet and go to a chatroom. The middle of the night for you is the middle of the day for someone else in the world. There are always people on-line to lend support.

In Your Notebook

Set up your support network to help you stay on track. Each day, write down some notes about how you can better use your support team to help stay on track. A notebook entry might look like this:

I was feeling at wit's end today, and I found myself eating lots of junk food as a result. To help prevent such situations, I can ask my friend Judy to help me by alternating days that we shuttle the kids to soccer practice. I can also ask my kids to pitch in by setting the table and washing the dishes after dinner.

Continue to monitor your hunger signals, trying to start eating at a 3 or 4 and stop by a 6 or 7 on the hunger scale.

Week 6: Reduce Temptations

Your last step to overcoming overeating is removing the final temptations that cause you to ignore your hunger signals. Here are some tips to help you:

• ELIMINATE PEER PRESSURE TO EAT. Be aware that some people will try to sabotage your weight-loss efforts. Some of these people will be easy to pinpoint. They are the ones who beg you to eat. "Come on, you're no fun anymore," they might tell you. Others are subtler. They might offer you food or encourage you to eat just by the fact that they are eating. They may not be conscious of their influence on you, but you need to be direct with them about what you do not want.
• PUT FOOD OUT OF SIGHT. Food can serve as a powerful cue to

eat. Have you ever found yourself eating after watching a television commercial about food? How about because you walked by the table and just happened to notice a bag of chips sitting on top of it? What about smells? Did you ever find yourself ordering fast food because the smell of the fries lured you in to the drive-through? Smells are so enticing that McDonald's and other food companies spend millions of dollars each year to develop artificial scents that increase food enjoyment. Fast food fries taste so good in part because they smell so good. Try to avoid such temptations, especially in the beginning stages of your weight-loss program. Put all food away so you can't see it. If a particular stretch of a road to and from work triggers the urge to eat, find another route. Do something else during television commercials. It's a healthy way of multitasking.

• WHEN YOU EAT, DO IT CONSCIOUSLY. Take your body off autopilot. Always sit down to eat, and turn off other distractions so you can tune in to your hunger. The TV and computer screen encourage you to tune out, so turn them off. Eat slowly so you can enjoy your food and feel satisfied. This will also help you avoid overeating because the hunger switch will get turned off before you overeat. Eliminating distractions will help you eat more slowly.

• EAT MINDFULLY. Tuning in to all of the smells, tastes, and sensations of eating will help slow you down and increase your enjoyment and satisfaction. It takes time for your stomach and brain to communicate feelings of satiety, so eat slowly. The faster you eat, the more likely you will eat too much food—suddenly going well past 7 on your hunger scale.

• BALANCE MONOTONY WITH VARIETY. We are hard-wired to eat when we see food, and studies show that we eat more when we see more. In particular, a large variety of food (such as a buffet) or a large amount of food (such as supersized restaurant portions) make us more likely to overeat. Avoid overstimulation when possible, particularly in the beginning of your weight-loss program.

On the other hand, you don't want to entirely avoid foods you like because that tends to trigger cravings. Thus, most of the time you don't want to have a lot of food choices available to you, and you certainly don't want to have unlimited amounts available to you. But you don't want to take all the pleasure out of eating. So when you do eat, eat good-quality, well-prepared foods that you like—and enjoy them. For example, treat yourself to fresh blueberries on your cereal every morning or buy really high quality oranges for your snacks instead of rice cakes.

As you get more in touch with your hunger cues, you might be able to test yourself by eating out at certain restaurants. But never beat yourself up for failure. At first, avoid tempting situations altogether, particularly places that serve large portion sizes and too much variety. When at home, you can mentally help yourself eat less and tune into hunger by serving smaller initial portions on a smaller-sized plate. You can always go back and get more—if you are still hungry.

In Your Notebook

Each day, pick a specific tempting situation, and jot down notes on ways you can overcome temptation. A notebook entry might look like this:

Today's tempting situation: Friends who encourage me to eat
Ways I can deal with this: (1) Explain to friends why overeating is so destructive to my health. (2) Meet friends only in non-food situations. (3) Minimize contact with those friends until I have more willpower and can firmly say no.

MIND-BODY EXERCISE

You can increase your chances of successfully starting and sticking with an exercise program by using your mind to your advantage. This isn't about willpower. This is about adopting habits that you find enjoyable and you can realistically stick with for the long haul. Here are some tips.

- FOCUS ON THE REWARDS, NOT THE DRAWBACKS. If you think that exercise is boring or too hard, you will not do it. Start by focusing on the health benefits. Also, try to add as many rewards to your exercise routine as possible. For example, walking with a friend allows you to look forward to the social nature of your exercise.

- EXPAND YOUR DEFINITION OF EXERCISE. You don't have to run, swim, or cycle to burn calories. Walking is a great form of exercise. Go for a walk before or after dinner. It will burn calories and help curb your appetite. Try ballroom or salsa dancing. Try chasing your kids or dog around the yard for a half-hour. As long as you make it fun, you'll be able to stick with it.

- REMOVE POSSIBLE OBSTACLES. Make exercise as convenient and inexpensive as possible. If you must drive forty-five minutes to the gym, you probably won't go very often. There are plenty of ways to exercise without leaving your home. Explore opportunities that will give you the lowest opportunity for coming up with excuses not to do it.

- TAKE A PERSONAL INVENTORY. Are you a social person, or do you prefer to be alone? If you're social, you may prefer a gym setting. If you like to keep to yourself, you'll probably enjoy home-based exercise. Similarly, some people enjoy only exercise that makes them sweat; others hate to sweat. Work with your natural tendencies, and choose a location, intensity, and exercise duration that best fit your personality and lifestyle.

11

From Caffeine to Valium

Substances That Affect Blood Sugar, Mind, and Body

MANY people, sometimes somewhat unconsciously, look to common everyday substances to regulate their moods. For example, to boost your mood and give yourself a jolt of energy in the morning or afternoon, you may turn to a cup of coffee. Or to help yourself calm down and release the stresses of a busy day, you may relax with a glass of wine or a beer. How about a cigarette to help you blow off steam after a heated argument? Others take this a step further, altering their moods with prescription medications, such as antidepressants and antianxiety medications to help calm their nervous systems. Still others use over-the-counter herbal supplements such as St. John's wort.

Many of these substances certainly help boost your mood, create energy, or help you calm down and release stress, but they're not all good for blood sugar. Indeed, some common over-the-counter and prescription drugs may worsen blood sugar. We scientists just don't know enough about some substances to say one way or the other.

Some medications can even influence whether you succeed on the Mind-Body Diabetes Revolution program. To help you improve your odds of success, I've provided a rundown of common over-the-counter and prescription drugs to help you work more effectively with your doctor to improve your mood while simultaneously improving your blood sugar control.

Let's start with the substance that just about every one of us has used at one time or another: caffeine.

Drug Interactions 101

In this chapter, I focus only on drugs that affect mood, but many other drugs interact with blood sugar control. For example, blood pressure medications such as beta-blockers and thiazide diuretics raise blood sugar. They are beyond the scope of this book. To find out more about such medications, consult your doctor.

CAFFEINE

Changing just one small morning habit can dramatically improve your results with the Mind-Body Diabetes Revolution program: give up your morning cup of coffee.

The caffeine in coffee that wakes you up in the morning also makes you more responsive to stress. Caffeine raises levels of the stress hormone epinephrine and also makes us more responsive to the epinephrine circulating in the bloodstream. As a result, your heart beats faster, your blood pressure increases, blood sugar rises—and you feel an initial jolt of energy. However, this jolt puts your body into fight-or-flight mode. According to research done by Dr. James Lane, one of my colleagues at Duke, drinking 1 cup of coffee in the morning can keep you in fight-or-flight mode until well into the evening. This research shows that four cups of coffee raises the hormone epinephrine by 32 percent all day long. Also, people who drink coffee report feeling more stressed throughout the day. Any outside stress, such as a frenzied day at work, will bump your epinephrine level even higher.

In short, caffeine makes you particularly sensitive to stress. If you scored high for hostility in Chapter 6, caffeine could determine whether you fly off the handle at a coworker who makes a mistake or whether you successfully handle the situation with assertiveness and ease. If you're prone to anxiety, your morning coffee may determine whether you suffer an anxiety attack as a deadline approaches or whether you can successfully talk yourself through the moment and stay on task.

This all spells trouble for blood sugar control. We've known for some years that caffeine can make cells resistant to insulin even in people who don't have diabetes. For example, in one study, researchers monitored the blood pressure, heart rate, and blood sugar for 2 hours after seven men took either a placebo or a caffeine pill. Caffeine increased insulin levels by 42 percent and decreased insulin sensitivity by 25 percent. Though blood sugar was roughly the same in all groups, none of the study subjects had diabetes.

In a recent study conducted by Dr. Lane, caffeine was just as bad in patients with type 2 diabetes. Fifteen patients who normally drank coffee volunteered to have their glucose tolerance measured before and after receiving either a dose of caffeine or a placebo. Caffeine clearly raised both the blood sugar and insulin of people with type 2 diabetes. This effect was greater in some people than in others, but on the average, caffeine negatively affected glucose tolerance.

Our results don't yet paint a black-and-white, open-and-shut case against caffeine. For example, we know that caffeine is probably bad for blood sugar, but we don't know if substances that contain caffeine, such as coffee and tea, affect blood sugar as adversely as pure caffeine. One study done on coffee found that it was associated with less risk for diabetes. The randomized study, completed in 2002 and published in the *Lancet,* followed more than 17,000 people for thirteen years. It compared coffee drinking to diabetes prevalence. Higher coffee consumption was associated with risk for a lot of unhealthy behaviors, including lack of exercise, smoking, and more body weight, but it wasn't associated with risk for type 2 diabetes. In fact, there seemed to be a protective effect.

How could this be? Here's one hypothesis. Coffee contains other substances beyond caffeine, such as chlorogenic acid and magnesium. These substances may offer protective effects for those with diabetes, counteracting the effects of caffeine on insulin sensitivity. Furthermore, it is possible that people who drink the most coffee may eat less than those who drink the least, thus helping them keep their weight down.

Tea provides another puzzle. Tea contains much less caffeine than coffee—30 milligrams per cup of tea compared to 100 or more milligrams per cup of coffee. Black, green, and white tea have also been shown to offer some heart disease protection. That's good because diabetes raises heart disease risk. But some emerging research shows that substances in green tea may boost the metabolism slightly. Though this boost might help you lose weight and subsequently improve your insulin sensitivity, we don't know if the metabolism boost in itself would adversely affect blood sugar control. To date, no research has looked directly at the effect of tea drinking on diabetes.

Exactly how caffeine affects your blood sugar may in part depend on your personality type and how much stress you are under. Caffeine magnifies stress significantly, which is why some people can drink a cup of coffee and go straight to bed: they already have such low stress levels that the coffee doesn't keep them awake. On the other hand, if you've already had a stressful day and drink a cup of coffee, you may remain awake for hours.

Caffeine may pose particular problems if you tested high for hostility in Chapter 6. Because caffeine stimulates the nervous system and because you are working to keep your nervous system calm, you greatly counteract the effects of the program by drinking caffeine. Your nervous system is already particularly sensitive, and you already react to stress in an exaggerated manner. Caffeine can make you even touchier. You may know someone who drinks six to seven cups of coffee a day and seems ready to explode at the slightest irritation. Also, if you already have a hard time turning off this stress response, caffeine may make your efforts even more difficult.

Caffeine appears to affect different people differently. To find out how it affects you, try this experiment. Check your blood sugar in the morning before breakfast. Then check it again 2 hours after you have eaten and had your morning coffee. Now switch to decaffeinated coffee for a week and also avoid soft drinks with caffeine. At the end of a week, repeat the blood sugar test with the same meal. Use an instant breakfast or Ensure both before and after you stop caffeine to help keep other possibly confounding factors constant. If you are sensitive to caffeine, your postmeal blood sugar will be lower after a week without caffeine. If you see no difference, then caffeine is probably not bothering you.

If you are sensitive to caffeine, you will want to give it up, and that isn't easy. It's almost an American birthright to use caffeine to boost productivity and performance. The vast majority of us reach for a cup of coffee or tea first thing in the morning. Caffeine helps keep us addicted because eventually we must drink caffeine to get to just a normal state of alertness and more and more of it to go beyond that. It wears off over time, and eventually you go through withdrawal if you don't have caffeine—withdrawal that includes headache, sleepiness, and moodiness. Also, if you're stressed, hostile, or depressed, you're already at a higher risk for caffeine dependency by nature of your mood or personality type.

Start with small steps. At first, you might try cutting back by a half-cup of coffee a day, or you might mix half decaffeinated and half caffeinated beans into your brew. Or, you might alternate a cup of coffee with a cup of tea, which contains much less caffeine. Keep working at it, and eventually you'll have lowered your dependence. Try to lower your caffeine consumption during a low-stress time at work and in the rest of your life.

NICOTINE

Many people turn to nicotine in times of stress. This couldn't be more counterproductive. But first, let me say that you should not beat yourself up over your dependence on whatever form of nicotine you choose. You've probably already been told time and again the list of reasons that you should quit. Becoming angry with yourself or depressed about your inability to quit may worsen your blood sugar control.

Nicotine is one of the most addictive substances around— even more addictive than heroin and cocaine. When you inhale smoke from a cigarette, the nicotine heads directly to your lungs, where small blood vessels absorb the drug into your blood, transporting it within seconds to your brain. Once there, nicotine produces many different effects, giving you a sense of calm, energy, and euphoria. Nicotine also increases blood pressure and heart rate, and possibly blood sugar as well. The effects of nicotine on the brain make you feel *really* good. Who wouldn't want to feel a surge of energy, calm, and clear thinking all at once? The problem is that it doesn't last. With each cigarette, it becomes harder and harder for you to reach that euphoric place. In fact, as soon as these brain chemical levels begin to fall, depression and fatigue follow, making you crave your next fix. You'll need more and more nicotine to produce the same reaction. If you go too long without nicotine, you enter withdrawal, feeling moody, lethargic, and confused.

Emerging research shows that some people are particularly prone to nicotine dependence. These same people are often also prone to depression, which nicotine temporarily lifts. That's why Zyban, a prescription antidepressant, has been used to help smokers kick the habit.

Now that you know why you smoke, let's take a look at four important reasons that you should quit:

1. Nicotine has been shown to constrict your blood vessels, which can decrease the absorption of injected insulin. In other words, it throws off the proper medication dosage that you need to shuttle blood sugar into cells.

2. Nicotine greatly raises your risk for heart disease. You're already at an increased risk because of your diabetes, and nicotine makes this even worse.

3. Though nicotine's effects on diabetes in particular are not well studied, it may worsen blood sugar control.

4. Nicotine causes your blood vessels to constrict, which makes you more likely to suffer a heart attack or stroke and can aggravate microvascular disease in your legs and elsewhere. Diabetes makes you more prone to developing damaged blood vessels. If you have compromised arteries, nicotine will aggravate the condition.

Surveys tell us that 60 to 90 percent of smokers relapse during their first year of trying to quit, but the encouraging news is that the more often you try to quit, the more likely you will quit.

Also, if you manage to make it a year without nicotine, your odds of staying nicotine free improve dramatically. Surveys show that only 15 percent of former smokers relapse during their second year of quitting, and only 2 to 4 percent relapse after two years.

To increase your chances of quitting, I recommend you try numerous strategies. Most important, don't do it alone. Because of nicotine's interaction with depression, I suggest you talk with your doctor about using Zyban to help you quit. Combine that with social support from your family, friends, the Internet, or a support group.

Your toughest period of withdrawal will come during the first two weeks off nicotine, so plan for this by quitting during a low-stress time period in your life—perhaps even by taking a vacation. Also, ask family members and friends to pitch in and help you with everyday tasks to lower your stress level. Finally, apologize in advance for how you may treat them during this time period. You *will* become grumpy, touchy, angry, or depressed during your withdrawal. Your relaxation techniques and cognitive behavior therapy program will also help you to navigate this period.

ALCOHOL

Of the trio of nonprescription substances that most of us turn to in times of stress, anger, or depression, alcohol poses the least risk of worsening blood sugar control. That does not make it completely benign, however.

Alcohol's effects on metabolism are complex. Alcohol has both a direct and indirect effect on caloric intake. Alcohol contains calories, and will increase your caloric intake and make you gain weight. Furthermore, alcohol is known to reduce inhibitions and stimulate your appetite. That's where the custom of having an aperitif before a meal came from. Research has shown that people who drink alcohol before a meal will eat more than if they don't have alcohol.

In contrast to caffeine and nicotine, alcohol can *lower* blood sugar. This isn't always better, particularly if you are already taking prescription diabetes medication to lower your blood sugar.

In people who don't have diabetes, the liver makes sugar only between meals. When they eat and their digested food consequently enters the bloodstream in the form of sugar, the liver senses a rise in insulin and turns off this sugar-making process. In people with diabetes, the liver doesn't correctly sense a rise in insulin—or the pancreas doesn't produce enough insulin— so the liver continues to make sugar even though the body doesn't need it. This is one of the problems that leads to high blood sugar. Your liver never turns off its sugar-making process.

Alcohol will turn off or turn down this process and seems to help lower this glucose production. If you take insulin or oral medications that increase your insulin secretion, however, alcohol may cause your blood sugar to drop too low. For example, many doctors tell their patients to take insulin right before bed in order to stop the liver from making sugar during the night. If you also have a drink or two before bed, you risk completely turning off the liver and having blood sugar drop too low.

This doesn't mean that you can't have a drink now and then, but it does mean that you must let your doctor know about it and work with your doctor to time your medication.

As far as heart health goes, alcohol seems to provide a protective effect. Numerous studies show that people who drink moderately—one to two drinks a day—have a lower risk of heart disease. None of these studies has looked at people with diabetes in particular, however. The studies have found that you must drink regularly and moderately to see an effect. Avoid splurging by consuming four or five drinks at a time. Spread out your consumption over the week—in one- to two-drink doses.

Drinking too much can damage the liver and raise blood pressure, both of which are already an issue for people with diabetes.

There's no reason that you must automatically exclude alcohol from your diet. Just keep your consumption moderate—no more than one to two drinks a day—and work with your doctor to time your consumption properly with your medication.

PRESCRIPTION ANTIDEPRESSANTS

Numerous prescription medications may help kick-start your brain in the right direction, helping to dramatically ease depression, anxiety, anger, or tension enough for you to complete this program successfully. Even better, many of these same medications may also help to lower your blood sugar levels.

But this isn't a black-and-white science. Drug treatment for people with diabetes is much trickier than for people who don't have diabetes because each drug poses a unique set of side effects that may either help or hinder blood sugar control. For example, if you are depressed, antidepressants may help, but you must make sure your doctor prescribes the right kind because some lower blood sugar and some raise it.

If you are depressed, and particularly if you have contemplated suicide, you may need prescription drugs to help lift your mood enough to tackle the program in this book and develop healthy habits such as exercise. Consider seeking professional attention and possibly antidepressant medications in addition to this program if your depression has lasted six months or longer, or if your depression is accompanied by severe symptoms, particularly suicidal thoughts. Some evidence shows that combining antidepressants with cognitive behavior therapy (such as the one suggested in this book) provides the best results in lifting depression.

Antidepressants lift depression in two out of three people who take them, usually achieving remission within three months. (The track record for psychotherapy is just as good. Consult Chapter 13 for tips on finding a good therapist.) Sometimes one drug may not work whereas another will, so be patient and work with your doctor to find the right antidepressant.

Antidepressants are also used to treat hostility syndrome, which is closely related to depression. But there's a big caveat here. There is a convincing amount of evidence about the link between stress and diabetes. Stress worsens blood sugar control, and relaxation—through the techniques described in this book or through antianxiety medications—improves it. We know less about depression, but enough to feel confident that depression leads to or worsens control of type 1 diabetes and that treating depression through therapy or through drugs probably helps improve blood sugar control in both types of diabetes. We know the least about hostility. We know that non-diabetic hostile people have minor abnormalities in glucose metabolism and may be at greater risk for developing diabetes. Scientists don't know, however, whether using drugs to treat hostility will help improve blood sugar control. That said, if you have such a severe anger problem that you can't even begin to think about attempting the techniques in this book, using anti-depressants may help you find the peace you need to get started.

No matter what type of antidepressant you try, take it for a few weeks to see if it works. Most of these drugs do not work overnight and need about two to four weeks to lift your mood. Antidepressants are not addictive, and you may need to remain on them for at least six months to a year's time.

Nearly all drugs pose at least some side effects, especially in the beginning. These include dry mouth, weight changes, and sexual dysfunction. Though most prescription drugs work at lifting mood, they don't all help improve blood sugar, and some hinder it. Consult the following list to help determine the pros and cons of different classes of antidepressants. Then work with your doctor to pinpoint the right class of medications for you.

- TRICYCLIC ANTIDEPRESSANTS. In addition to lifting depression, this class of antidepressants, such as nortriptyline (Aventyl), amitriptyline (Elavil), and imipramine (Tofranil), excel at helping to relieve insomnia and reduce pain. On the down-side, they tend to result in weight gain, which can worsen insulin resistance in people with diabetes. A recent study by Dr. Patrick Lustman at Washington University found that one of these drugs, nortriptyline, raised blood sugar even when those taking it didn't gain weight. These drugs also tend to worsen heart health, making them a poor choice for those who already have heart disease as a result of diabetes. For these reasons, I recommend avoiding this class of antidepressants altogether if you have diabetes.
- SELECTIVE SEROTONIN REUPTAKE INHIBITORS (SSRIs). You probably know this class of drugs better by the brand name Prozac (flu-

oxetine). Other brand names are Zoloft (sertraline), Paxil (paroxetine), and Effexor (venlafaxine). Unlike tricyclic antidepressants, this class of medications was thought for many years to improve blood sugar control in most people with diabetes without causing weight gain. For many years, they have been the antidepressants of choice for people with diabetes. This class of antidepressants is also most often used to treat hostility syndrome.

New evidence suggests that these drugs may not be as benign as we once thought. Very recent data suggest that these drugs may promote weight gain, at least in some people. While they are probably okay, you need to work with your doctor to monitor your blood sugar and weight while taking them.

In certain people with diabetes, these drugs may not be a good idea. SSRIs tend to cause gastrointestinal distress. If your diabetes already is causing that complication, SSRIs will probably worsen the problem. Most of these drugs can inhibit orgasm during sex. Since sexual problems are common in patients with diabetes, this side effect can make a bad situation worse.

- **WELLBUTRIN AND ZYBAN.** These drugs contain bupropion hydrochloride. Unlike other types of antidepressants, bupropion does not have sexual side effects, and it may actually induce weight loss. In one study published in *Obesity Research* in 2002, depressed obese adults who received bupropion while also cutting calories lost more weight than those who didn't receive the drug. Bupropion's effect on weight loss probably improves insulin sensitivity. It is probably a good choice for people with diabetes.

  This antidepressant has also been proved helpful in those trying to quit smoking. Bupropion is marketed as Zyban for the treatment of nicotine addiction. As you wean yourself off nicotine, the brain chemical dopamine will fall, causing anxiety and depression. Zyban may counteract this dopamine drop, helping to ease the psychological ramifications of quitting, as well as weight gain.

However, even this class of medications may not be good for everyone. Consult your physician to see if bupropion may be helpful for you.

• ESTROGEN REPLACEMENT THERAPY. You wouldn't normally think of estrogen replacement therapy (ERT) as a first choice treatment for lifting depression. However, women who go through menopause often also feel depressed, and some research shows ERT helps lift that depression. Also, a very well-designed study published in the *British Medical Journal* in 2003 found that women who took ERT at menopause were less likely to develop diabetes after menopause. We know from animal studies that estrogen somehow counteracts diabetes. In fact, we usually study only male animals because the females often don't develop diabetes.

The same is true in humans. Women often don't develop diabetes until after menopause. They may become insulin resistant before menopause, but full-blown diabetes usually doesn't develop until estrogen levels drop.

Of course, ERT is controversial for many reasons, including its link with an increased risk for breast cancer, heart disease, and Alzheimer's disease. Talk with your doctor about your personal health history to weigh your individual pros and cons for ERT.

Herbal Remedies

One herb has gained much popularity over the years in the treatment of depression: St John's wort. Little is known about how this herb interacts with blood sugar control, though St. John's wort is already known to interact negatively with cancer, heart disease, birth control, and AIDs drugs. It has many of the same side effects as tricyclic antidepressants and therefore should probably be avoided in people with diabetes.

More startling is the fact that the herb may not hold up to its promise. In a recent trial conducted at Duke and sponsored by the National Institutes of Health, St. John's wort was no more effective than a placebo (sugar pill) for treating major depression.

I strongly suggest staying away from herbal remedies. Although some of them may be helpful, they are not as well studied as prescription drugs. We just don't know how they affect blood sugar.

ANTIANXIETY MEDICATION

Some antianxiety medications offer beneficial effects on blood sugar. A class of antianxiety medications called benzodiazepines (which includes Xanax and Valium) has been shown in studies with both humans and animals to lower blood sugar over the short term.

They may do this in two ways: by lowering levels of stress hormones or by somehow acting directly on the pancreas. Benzodiazepine receptors on the pancreas may help stimulate insulin release, so these drugs may act directly on metabolic function.

Using medications to treat anxiety is controversial, particularly because most types of antianxiety medications are habit forming. They all make you feel pleasantly calm, but over time, you develop a tolerance and need more and more medication to arrive at the same effect. When you don't take them, you experience withdrawal symptoms. That's why you should not take such drugs longer than three weeks.

The good news is that you don't have to. Progressive muscle relaxation works just as well as prescription tranquilizers at lowering anxiety and normalizing blood sugar. In a study that I and others at Duke did during the 1990s, we found a significant link between a patient's response to Xanax and his or her response to progressive muscle relaxation. In other words, if Xanax helped lower their blood sugar, progressive muscle relaxation did as well. Progressive muscle relaxation gives the effect of the drug *without* the drug.

Nevertheless, there are two situations that may merit using a tranquilizer. First, if you are so anxious that you can't even begin to tackle the program, a short course of these drugs may be helpful. Second, if you need a little personal proof that the mind-body program in this book will improve your blood sugar control, a short course of these drugs may help you to see the light.

Because antianxiety medications lower blood sugar just as well as progressive muscle relaxation, you can take them for two weeks to see if they have an effect. If your blood sugar goes down, you can rest assured that you can keep it down by tackling the progressive muscle relaxation program in Chapter 7.

OVER-THE-COUNTER DRUGS

Besides caffeine, nicotine, and some prescription drugs, certain over-the-counter medications and supplements may adversely affect diabetes by triggering the fight-or-flight response. When shopping for medicines, examine the label, and always check to see if it lists diabetes as a contraindication. Also, check with your pharmacist to see if the drug is contraindicated for diabetes.

A few over-the-counter medicines known to aggravate diabetes include these:

• ANTIHISTAMINES. In addition to hindering blood sugar metabolism, antihistamines can increase appetite if used chronically, causing weight gain that can worsen blood sugar control.

• DECONGESTANTS. The labels of most over-the-counter decongestants used for colds have a warning about using these medications if you have diabetes. The reason is that most of these remedies contain phenylephrine, a close relative of epinephrine. Epinephrine is a stress hormone that will release stored blood sugar. If possible, avoid these drugs.

• FAT BURNERS. Emerging research shows that supplements that contain a combination of ephedra and caffeine speed the metabolism and result in weight loss. Weight loss should improve your insulin sensitivity, but these drugs are not the answer. We don't know how these supplements affect blood sugar over the short term. Also, the Food and Drug Administration has linked more than seventy bad reactions, including death, to these supplements. Because diabetes raises your risk for heart disease and other health problems, you're particularly prone to these negative interactions. Don't take fat burners.

GOOD EXCITEMENT

I mentioned earlier in the book that your body doesn't have the ability to recognize the difference between good and bad stress. It responds to both with a rise in stress hormones. Yet you don't always want to immunize yourself from stress. For example, few of us would want to feel blissfully calm during a birthday party or some other celebration. Sexual intercourse also raises stress hormone levels. Do you need to practice progressive muscle relaxation before sex? No.

To deal better with "good stress," work with your doctor to time your diabetes medications correctly. I can't give you a formula to follow in order to use medication to help your body to counter the effects of excitement. You'll need to work with your doctor to do that. But know that you are allowed and even encouraged to feel excitement.

12

The Wide World of Relaxation

Six Additional Mind-Body Techniques

PROGRESSIVE muscle relaxation is the simplest, easiest to learn, and most practical way to relax, and the one that has been directly proven to help control blood sugar in diabetes, but it's certainly not the only way to relax. If you have difficulty with progressive muscle relaxation, you can experiment with other relaxation methods. Even if you love progressive muscle relaxation, you may decide to incorporate more than one method into your lifestyle. For example, you might decide to use progressive muscle relaxation throughout the day to relax at work and a different technique at night to help wind down for sleep or to make the transition from the stress at work to a more calming atmosphere at home. It just depends on your needs.

In this chapter, we look at five other techniques that have received positive attention from researchers over the years. Experiment with any or all to see which ones work best for you.

TRANSCENDENTAL MEDITATION

There are many different forms of meditation. Some schools of meditation encourage you to focus on your breath. Others use prayers, single words or phrases, and religious devotions to quiet the mind. Still others strive to quiet the mind, eliminating every thought until the mind is a blank slate, whereas others focus on noticing your thoughts and turning inward.

Transcendental meditation (TM) was introduced to the United States from India by Maharishi Mahesh Yogi and popularized by Harvard physician Herbert Benson in his bestselling book *The Relaxation Response* (1975). Perhaps the most studied form of meditation, TM has had more than 500 studies completed on its effects on blood pressure, heart rate, and blood sugar.

Maharishi Mahesh Yogi markets the technique through his Maharishi University of Management in Fairfield, Iowa. At the university, as well as some sites around the country, meditation students receive a specific mantra customized to their body types. During meditation, the practitioner silently repeats his or her mantra over and over to quiet and calm mind chatter.

Benson probably would not have studied TM had it not been for a group of very persistent students who had learned it and claimed that they could lower their blood pressure through meditation. Eventually, he decided to study his students and fitted them with devices to measure their breathing rate, brain waves, and other bodily functions. He was surprised by the results. During meditation, the students consumed 17 percent less oxygen. Their breathing rate slowed from fourteen to fifteen breaths per minute to ten to eleven breaths per minute, and their lactate levels dropped in the bloodstream, an indication of calm and tranquility. Brain wave patterns slowed.

Benson has since performed numerous other studies that show the health benefits of TM. Most of his subsequent experiments to test TM were done on blood pressure. In one, thirty-six people had their blood pressure measured for six weeks, and then they learned to practice TM for two weeks. Their blood pressure was measured several times a day but not during meditation. The participants' average blood pressure dropped from systolic 146 to 137, lowering them from high to borderline normal. Diastolic dropped from 93.5 to 88.9, again lowering average pressure from high to borderline normal.

Benson's research has shown that focusing the mind on any object, word, or phrase will elicit the same deep inner calm. If you've ever felt peaceful after performing a religious chant, ritual, or repetitious prayer such as the Rosary, you've experienced the effects of TM. The repetition of the word or phrase helps cancel out other thoughts, calm your mind, and bring you to a peaceful state.

Although TM certainly results in a deep sense of calm, it's hard to do anyplace, anytime. When you're in a heated discussion with your boss, you don't want to tell your boss, "Hold on while I close my eyes, breathe deeply, and concentrate on my mantra." Indeed, Benson's studies show that TM boosts health only as long as you practice it regularly. As soon as practitioners stopped meditating, their blood pressure rose.

Here are some pointers for starting a TM-type practice:

- Meditate in a quiet room. Sit comfortably during a time of day when you are not fatigued and won't be easily distracted.
- Before you start, pick a mantra—a one-syllable word to recite mentally to yourself, such as *one, peace,* or *love.*
- Close your eyes.
- Calm your mind by focusing on your breathing. Breathe in and out through your nose, noticing the rise and fall of your abdomen with every breath. Listen to the sound of your breath and feel the sensation of breath coming in through your nose and lungs.
- Relax all of your muscles, starting at your feet and moving up toward your neck, forehead, and face.
- Continue to breathe easily and naturally through your nose. Don't force your breath.
- As you exhale, mentally say your mantra to yourself. Focus on your mantra on each exhalation for 10 to 20 minutes.
- Disregard any intrusive thoughts. When something else enters your mind, silently say, "No" or "Oh." Let distracting thoughts pass like clouds, and return your focus to your mantra.
- Don't worry about how well you are doing. Resist the urge to evaluate your performance.
- When you are finished, sit quietly for a few moments. Don't race back to life's hassles.

RELAXATION AND EXERCISE

Physical exercise may help you control your blood sugar in more ways than one. You may know that exercise conditions lean muscle tissue, which helps to make your muscle cells more sensitive to the uptake of sugar. It also tends to relax you and helps you to obliterate stress.

You may be able to magnify this stress-reducing effect of exercise by meditating as you move. During the late 1970s, Herbert Benson asked exercisers to focus on a word, phrase, prayer, or some other mantra as they cycled on stationary bikes. He had a control group of other cyclists who performed the same amount of exercise but without a mantra. Those who focused on the mantra disregarded other thoughts, basically meditating while moving. They slowed their metabolic rates by 11 percent compared to those who didn't focus on a mantra.

The next time you power walk, run, cycle, or swim, create a moving meditation. You could focus on your breathing as you exercise: as you inhale, silently say *in,* and as you exhale, silently say *out.* Or you might silently repeat "one, two, three" as your feet hit the ground.

QIGONG

Qigong (pronounced "chee gung"), which originated in China, combines deep, controlled breathing with slow body movements. In English, *Qi* translates to "energy." The Chinese have long believed that this ancient energy practice can heal and prevent everything from high blood pressure to depression and heart disease.

It appears the practice may also help improve blood sugar control in people with type 2 diabetes. A recent study published in *Diabetes Care* split thirty-six patients with type 2 diabetes into two groups. The first group underwent four months of Qigong training whereas the second group did not. After 4 months, HbA_{1C} levels, a measure of long-term blood sugar control, improved 0.8 percent. That may not sound like much, but it's a significant improvement—as good as or better than many diabetes medications.

Though Qigong involves body movements that could improve blood sugar control by conditioning muscles, the researchers who conducted the study suspect that practitioners received the most benefit from the deep sense of relaxation that Qigong provides. To learn Qigong, you will need to take a class from a qualified instructor. To find a class near you, go to www.qi.org or www.npa.org.

AUTOGENIC TRAINING

I became familiar with autogenic training, a form of self-hypnosis, during the late 1970s, when I was researching how to use the mind-body connection to help patients with Raynaud's disease to warm their hands and feet, dramatically improving their quality of life. Because it deeply relaxes the body, it will also help you turn on your parasympathetic nervous system and *possibly* improve blood sugar control.

Autogenic training was developed by a German neurologist named Dr. H. H. Shultz during the early 1900s. Shultz had heard stories about a pharmacist named Emile Coué who taught affirmations (positive self-talk) to his patients at a free clinic in the early 1900s. Coué told his patients to repeat, "Every day in every way, I am getting better and better," twenty times to themselves every day. Intrigued, Shultz developed a specific set of affirmations in the 1930s designed to relax the body. The affirmations used the words *heavy* and *warm*. Psychologists believe that suggestions of the sensations of heaviness release muscle tension, and thoughts and sensations of warmth increase blood flow to the muscles. These affirmations have been shown to help those with Raynaud's warm their hands and feet. They have not been studied in people with diabetes, but they probably work by inducing the relaxation response.

The sympathetic nervous system is closely related to our emotions, how warm we feel, skin temperature, and internal body temperature. When the sympathetic nervous system is active due to the fight-or-flight response, blood vessels constrict and cause blood flow to the hands and feet to decrease. That makes you feel cold, but your body is actually conserving heat. When you are hot, blood vessels in your fingers and toes dilate to release the heat. When you are cold, they constrict to hold in heat. This is why rings may feel tighter on a hot day—the dilated blood vessels cause your fingers to swell. In someone with Raynaud's disease, this response to temperature is exaggerated, so autogenic training helps activate the relaxation response and allows the person to focus on sensations of warmth.

Like progressive muscle relaxation, autogenic training results in a state of deep relaxation. As with progressive muscle relaxation, you must practice autogenic training several times a day until you can relax automatically. Start with two 15-minute sessions. Make sure the room is no colder than 75 degrees, or your efforts will be more difficult. If you keep your house cooler than that, practice in the bathroom just after taking a shower, or use a small space heater.

You'll need a small, comfortable chair that allows you to relax with your arms resting on your knees and your head bending slightly forward. This position will help increase blood flow to the hands. Use this body position until you can consistently warm your hands.

To practice autogenic training, read the script that follows into a tape or digital recorder. Then play it back to yourself during your sessions. If you don't like the sound of your own voice, ask someone else to read the instructions into the recorder.

Start each session by getting comfortable and relaxing by focusing on your breathing. Notice sensations of pulsing warmth in your fingers. At the end of your session, open your eyes, and reorient yourself to your surroundings.

Script for Autogenic Training

Read the following script into a tape or digital recorder. Talk slowly and softly. Pause where indicated for the specified amount of time, but don't say the word _pause_ into the recorder. Simply stop talking and remain quiet. You will need a long pause on your tape after you finish the instructions and before you say your last line. So make sure to run the tape recorder in a quiet room to avoid capturing distracting sounds on the tape.

This script focuses on teaching you to relax by making your hands feel heavy. Once you feel comfortable with the technique, you can take it a step further. Make another tape, but this time substitute the words *warm* and *heavy* instead of *heavy* and *relaxed*. Feelings of heaviness are easier to achieve than feelings of warmth. Once you've mastered feelings of heaviness, you're ready for this additional challenge. Because increasing blood flow will make you feel warmer and because increasing blood flow is indicative of decreasing sympathetic nervous system activity, increasing warmth is a better indicator of your control over the fight-or-flight response.

I feel quite quiet.

PAUSE 10 SECONDS

I am beginning to feel quite relaxed.

PAUSE 10 SECONDS

My right foot feels heavy and relaxed.

PAUSE 10 SECONDS

My left foot feels heavy and relaxed.

PAUSE 10 SECONDS

My ankles, knees, and hips feel heavy, relaxed, and comfortable.

PAUSE 10 SECONDS

My abdomen and chest feel heavy and relaxed.

PAUSE 10 SECONDS

My neck, jaw, and forehead feel completely relaxed.

PAUSE 10 SECONDS

They feel comfortable and smooth.

PAUSE 10 SECONDS

My right arm feels heavy and relaxed.

PAUSE 10 SECONDS

My left arm feels heavy and relaxed.

PAUSE 10 SECONDS

My right hand feels heavy and relaxed.

PAUSE 10 SECONDS

My left hand feels heavy and relaxed.

PAUSE 10 SECONDS

Both of my hands feel heavy and relaxed.

PAUSE 10 SECONDS

Repeat to yourself silently, "My hands feel heavy and relaxed."

PAUSE 10 SECONDS

My hands feel heavy and relaxed.

PAUSE 10 SECONDS

Stop reciting the phrases, and slowly allow yourself to reorient to the room. You may open your eyes and stand up when you are ready.

MINDFULNESS MEDITATION

Part of a type of meditation called *vipassana,* or insight meditation, mindfulness meditation comes from Buddhist traditions and is more than 2,500 years old. It was popularized during the 1970s by a Harvard researcher, Jon Kabat-Zinn, Ph.D., who has since moved on to the Stress Reduction Clinic at the University of Massachusetts Medical Center, where he continues to teach the technique.

In this form of meditation, you focus your attention fully on an activity at hand, such as eating, walking, sitting in the sun, listening to music, or even washing the dishes. You can also practice this form of meditation with your eyes closed by focusing your mindfulness inward, noticing bodily sensations, the act of breathing, your thoughts, your feelings, even discomfort.

Kabat-Zinn and other proponents say that mindfulness balances the body and mind and gives practitioners a greater awareness that helps them to deal with life's problems. Kabat-Zinn has found that mindfulness, like other relaxation methods, can elicit the relaxation response to help achieve better health, and he has taught the technique to thousands of people with a wide range of medical ailments. Although the technique is much less studied than TM, anecdotal reports offer encouragement that it probably produces the same health effects.

One recent study found that mindfulness meditation worked as well as therapy at lowering stress-related symptoms. Others have found that it helps to decrease pain, improve the skin condition psoriasis, reduce anxiety, and decrease fibromyalgia discomfort. One study even found a reduction in the number of doctor's visits among those who practiced this form of meditation.

Unlike TM, you can use mindfulness meditation when you are caught in a stressful situation. You don't need to close your eyes to practice. Rather, you need only observe your actions and situation with your full attention, as if you were watching yourself from afar. This detachment helps soothe feelings of anger, stress, and anxiety. You simply acknowledge the present moment, good or bad.

Here are some pointers for developing a mindful meditation practice:

- Commit forty-five minutes, six days a week to the technique.
- Keep an open mind. If you think that it won't do anything, then you won't have the discipline to stick with it. You don't have to like doing it, but you must remain open. Don't expect anything to happen or not to happen. Just try it for a couple of weeks.
- Calm yourself by taking three deep breaths slowly.
- Pick something to devote your attention to.
- Notice the smells, sounds, sensations, tastes, colors, shapes, feelings, and so on. Use every sense to experience the moment.
- When thoughts pop up, acknowledge them. You are not psychoanalyzing yourself, but you are also not chasing your thoughts away. Don't judge yourself. Just notice your thoughts as they pass through your mind.
- Accept your feelings, emotions, thoughts, and sensations for what they are. This will make you more aware and in touch with what is happening to you and in you.

Turning Your Focus Inward

You can meditate mindfully by turning your focus inward and experiencing every aspect of your inner being. To do so, follow these steps:

1. Lie on your back in a comfortable position.
2. Close your eyes.
3. Notice your breath. Smell it, feel it, and experience it.

4. Slowly move your attention to various aspects of your body. Start at your feet, and move upward toward your head. Notice any sensations. Some sensations may feel good, others bad, others neutral. Notice sensations of warmth and coolness. Notice sensations of tightness or openness.

5. Imagine breathing into any areas of discomfort. For example, if your calf feels tight, mentally breathe into it with every exhalation. If you feel sad or angry, imagine breathing into your heart.

6. Imagine inhaling your breath through the bottom of your feet. Imagine the breath traveling up your body. Then exhale, and imagine it leaving through the crown of your head.

7. Finish by spending a few moments noticing whatever drifts in and out of your awareness.

Living in the Moment

You can meditate mindfully anywhere you find yourself by bringing your mind fully to the present moment. Often, we spend many of our waking hours living in the past or future. If you've ever driven somewhere and don't actually remember the trip, then you know what I mean.

For brief periods of time, try fully bringing your attention to somewhat mundane tasks, such as eating or cleaning. Use your eyes, ears, nose, mouth, and skin to give yourself information about what you are experiencing. For example, while eating, notice the color of your food. Notice the texture and taste as you chew it. Notice how it feels when you swallow. Notice the changing sensations in your stomach from empty to full. These brief periods of meditation will help tune you in to some of the greatest joys in life, many of which you would otherwise have missed by traveling the earth on autopilot.

DISCLOSURE THERAPY

The psychologist James Pennenbaker discovered that simply expressing your emotional thoughts in writing can be extremely therapeutic. He called this technique *self-disclosure therapy,* meaning that the disclosure is simply made to yourself. The idea is that if you can spill out your deepest feelings, especially those concerning stress and trauma, you will, in the process, develop coping skills.

I discovered the stress-reducing benefits of disclosure therapy not long ago, when my wife was diagnosed with breast cancer. From her diagnosis to treatment to recovery, I felt just about every emotion you can name, from sadness to anger to fear to depression. Yet I felt I couldn't talk to my wife about some of these feelings because I wanted to be strong for her. I wanted to do what I could to help her through the ordeal. So I turned to journaling. Each day I sat down in front of my computer and typed out my thoughts and feelings. After typing up everything that came to mind, I felt more relaxed and able to handle our situation. After a mastectomy and chemotherapy, Sandra is now in remission, and our marriage is as strong and close as ever. I thank disclosure therapy for much of that.

Disclosure therapy involves nothing more than writing down your thoughts and feelings. You don't need to tell anyone else, just yourself. Though we have not studied the effects of this practice on diabetes, we do know that disclosure therapy helps relieve stress in other conditions. For example, one study of forty-five people over age sixty-five found that three twenty-minute daily writing sessions resulted in a significant decrease in doctor's visits. Other research has found that self-disclosure can help improve lung function in patients with asthma and reduce pain in those with arthritis.

Disclosure therapy is thought to help you to release your grip on negative thoughts. Any time we bottle up negative thoughts, we spend a great deal of mental energy and activate the autonomic nervous system. Releasing those thoughts helps you organize your feelings, allows you to understand them, and often helps you uncover solutions. You gain a sense of control over your problem.

There is no right or wrong way to do it. Simply sit down at a computer keyboard or typewriter, pick up a pen and paper, or use a tape recorder, and allow your inner thoughts to spill out. In particular, the therapy helps you deal with distressing thoughts, events, or emotions such as anger.

You can use self-disclosure to revisit old problems or events from earlier in your life. Think back to a distressing life experience, and then write down your thoughts and emotions associated with it. These might involve relationships with others. How have they affected your past, present, or future? How do you see the people and events now, differently from in the past?

Some researchers believe that you must share your self-disclosure with another person for the method to be most effective. That may help because it can deepen your relationships with others, and a wealth of research shows that social contacts are important to well-being. Sharing it with others also allows you to receive feedback from them about your opinions and thoughts, allowing some objectivity in your feelings. A wealth of research shows that sharing your emotions with others will improve your health.

Here are some pointers for using disclosure therapy to reduce stress:

- Set aside a time of day to write about your thoughts. Pick a time when you won't feel rushed.
- Think back over your day. When did you feel angry, rushed, stressed, or sad? Write about this event and any feelings associated with it.
- Try to write a few sentences with the words *because, reason, understand,* and *realize.* These words will help you to come to some conclusions about what you've written.
- Don't judge your writing. Just allow it to spill out.

A PERSONAL PREFERENCE

As you can see, there are many different ways to manage stress. Use progressive muscle relaxation as the cornerstone in your relaxation plan. You can do that anywhere at any time. Then if you wish, experiment with the different ways to relax suggested in this chapter as you see fit. The more you practice, the more natural relaxation becomes. Eventually, relaxation will become an integral part of your life—as natural as getting up in the morning and brushing your teeth.

13
Getting More Help

Resources to Help You Maximize the Program

I'd love to promise that this book will help every person with diabetes reduce stress, lift depression and hostility, diminish overeating, improve blood sugar control, and achieve a better life, but some readers may need more than just this book to see results. For some people who are suffering from acute stress, depression, or hostility, seeking professional help from a therapist, psychologist, or psychiatrist may be a better first step than trying to work alone. For others, professional advice along with the advice in this book may provide the perfect treatment.

Who should seek help and who can safely tackle the program alone? The answer to that question is not an easy one, but here are some signals that you may need professional help:

- You've tried the tips and programs in this book for six weeks and continue to feel just as depressed, stressed, anxious, or hostile.
- You are contemplating or have contemplated suicide.
- You'd like to try the program but can't seem to find the motivation to get started.
- You are already seeing a therapist. There's no reason to stop just because you have this book. Discuss the methods suggested in the book with your therapist.
- You are so anxious, depressed, or hostile that you no longer

can function normally. For example, you no longer go to work, you turn down all social engagements, and you spend the majority of each day in bed.

If you decide to seek professional help, this doesn't make you a failure. Consulting a mental health professional to get your stress, mood, or hostility under control is similar to consulting a diabetes specialist about your diabetes. Don't be ashamed to do so. Remember that deciding to seek help means that you are taking a proactive step for your emotional and physical health. Seeking out help requires courage. Congratulate yourself on making a firm commitment to getting as much help as you can to improve your health.

This chapter contains tips on finding the best therapist for you. It also lists key contacts for finding out more about various mind-body therapies mentioned throughout this book, such as transcendental and mindfulness meditation.

CHOOSING A THERAPIST

Most important in choosing a therapist is the chemistry between you and your therapist. You must feel comfortable. You should feel as if you connect. You should feel safe revealing your innermost secrets. You should be able to trust that your sessions and what you reveal will be kept private.

To find a therapist, you might ask for a referral from your family doctor or endocrinologist. You can also contact the following organizations, all of which offer "find a therapist" options on their websites:

American Diabetes Association
1701 North Beauregard Street
Alexandria, VA 22311
800-DIABETES
http://www.diabetes.org/

American Psychiatric Association
1000 Wilson Boulevard, Suite 1825

Arlington, VA 22209-3901
888-35-PSYCH or 703-907-7300
Fax: 703-907-7322
http://www.psych.org

American Psychological Association
750 First Street, NE
Washington, DC 20002-4242
800-374-2721 or 202-336-5500
http://www.apa.org

Association for the Advancement of Behavior Therapy
305 Seventh Avenue, 16th Floor
New York, NY 10001-6008
212-647-1890
Fax: 212-647-1865
http://www.aabt.org

National Association of Cognitive-Behavior Therapists
NACBT
P.O. Box 2195
Weirton, WV 26062
800-853-1135
Outside the U.S.: 304-723-3982
http://www.nacbt.org
Email: nacbt@nacbt.org

National Registry of Licensed Psychotherapists
http://www.psychotherapistsearch.com

Society for Behavioral Medicine
7600 Terrace Avenue, Suite 203
Middleton, WI 53562
608-827-7267
Fax: 608-831-5485
http://www.sbmweb.org
Email: info@sbmweb.org

PROGRAMS AND SUPPORT

In addition to or in lieu of working one-on-one with a therapist, you may find it helpful to explore further training in the various relaxation techniques described in Chapters 7, 10, and 13. Here are some resources to help you in your quest for more information and fine-tuning:

Transcendental Meditation

Maharishi University of Management
1000 North Fourth Street
Fairfield, Iowa 52557
800-369-6480 OR 641-472-1110
http://www.tm.org OR www.mum.org
Email: info@tm.org

Mind/Body Medical Institute
824 Boylston Street
Chestnut Hill, MA 02467
617-991-0102 or 866-509-0732
Fax: 617-991-0112
http://www.mbmi.org
Email: MBMI@CareGroup.Harvard.edu

Mindfulness Meditation

Center for Mindfulness at the University of Massachusetts
55 Lake Avenue
North Worcester, MA 01605
http://www.umassmed.edu/cfm
Email: mindfulness@umassmed.edu

Duke Center for Integrative Medicine
P.O. Box 3022
Duke University Medical Center
Durham, NC 27710
919-660-6745
http://www.dcim.org

Stress Management

Department of Psychiatry and Behavioral Sciences
Duke University Medical Center
Durham, NC 27710
919-684-0100
http://psychiatry.mc.duke.edu

Biofeedback

Association for Applied Psychophysiology
    and Biofeedback
10200 West 44th Avenue, Suite 304
Wheat Ridge, CO 80033-2840
303-422-8436
Fax: 303-422-8894
http://www.aapb.org
Email: aapb@resourcenter.com

Biofeedback Network
125 Prospect Street
Phoenixville, PA 19460
610-933-8145
Fax: 610-983-9162
http://www.biofeedback.net
Email: miller@biofeedback.net

Weight Loss

Duke Diet and Fitness Center
800-235-3853
Fax: 919-684-8246
Email: dfcinfo@dukecenter.org

Rice Diet Program
Rice House
1644 Cole Mill Road
Durham, NC 27705
919-383-7276 ext. 2
http://www.ricedietprogram.com

Structure House
3017 Picket Road
Durham, NC 27710
919-493-4205
http://www.structurehouse.com

HELP WITH LIFESTYLE CHANGES

In the previous chapter, you learned how smoking raises your risk for heart disease. If you'd like to quit, don't go it alone. Research shows that support, from friends or even on-line, can help you better navigate the toughest first few weeks of your nicotine-free lifestyle.

For help, try any of the following:

- For on-line support and information: www.quitnet.com
- To download the surgeon general's tobacco cessation guide: www.surgeongeneral.gov/tobacco/default.htm
- For information about smoking and quitting and to find a support group near you: the American Lung Association's website at www.lungusa.org/tobacco
- For a list of on-line support groups: www.whyquit.com

GENERAL INFORMATION

The more you know about diabetes, the better you'll be able to deal with the disease. Here are some ways to learn more:

If you don't already have an endocrinologist, contact the American Association of Clinical Endocrinologists for a referral. The website offers a membership directory.

American Association of Clinical Endocrinologists
1000 Riverside Avenue, Suite 205
Jacksonville, FL 32204
904-353-7878
Fax: 904-353-8185
http://www.aace.com

To find out more about drug interactions, download a free pamphlet from the Food and Drug Administration (http://vm

.cfsan.fda.gov/~lrd/fdinter.html) or go to the Express Scripts DrugDigest(http://www.drugdigest.org/DD/Interaction/ChooseDrugs). When in doubt ask your physician or pharmacist.

For general information about diabetes, contact the American Diabetes Association, the nation's leading nonprofit diabetes organization devoted to research, advocacy, and information. Its website offers basic information about almost anything you could ever want to know about diabetes.

> National Call Center
> 1701 North Beauregard Street
> Alexandria, VA 22311
> 800-DIABETES
> http://www.diabetes.org

For information on following a healthy diet or for a referral on a registered dietician in your area, contact the American Dietetic Association.

> 800/366-1655
> http://www.eatright.org

FURTHER READING

To learn more about mind-body techniques and health, consult the following books:

Benson, Herbert, *The Relaxation Response* (New York: Morrow, 1975)

———, *Beyond the Relaxation Response* (New York: Times Books, 1984)

Greenberger, Dennis, and Padesky, Christine, *Mind over Mood* (New York: Guilford Press, 1995)

Williams, Redford, *The Trusting Heart* (New York: Times Books, 1989)

Williams, Redford, and Williams, Virginia, *Anger Kills* (New York: Times Books, 1993)

Selected Bibliography

STRESS

Surwit, R. S., et al. (1984). "Behavioral manipulation of the diabetic pheno-type in ob/ob mice." *Diabetes,* vol. 33, pp. 616–618.

Surwit, R., et al. (1985). "Classically conditioned hyperglycemia in the obese mouse." *Psychosomatic Medicine,* vol. 47, no. 6, pp. 565–568.

Surwit, R. S., et al. (1988). "Diet-induced type II diabetes in C57BL/6J mice." *Diabetes,* vol. 37, pp. 1163–1167.

Surwit, R. S. (1993). "Of mice and men: Behavioral medicine in the study of type II diabetes." *Annals of Behavioral Medicine,* vol. 15, no. 4, pp. 227–235.

Surwit, R. S., et al. (1993). "Role of stress in the etiology and treatment of diabetes mellitus." *Psychosomatic Medicine,* vol. 55, pp. 380–393.

Surwit, R. S., et al. (1994). "Glycemic response to stress is altered in eu-glycemic Pima Indians." *International Journal of Obesity,* vol. 18, no. 11, pp. 766–770.

Surwit, R. S., et al. (1996). "Animal models provide insight into psychoso-matic factors in diabetes." *Psychosomatic Medicine,* vol. 58, pp. 582–589.

DEPRESSION

Clouse, R. E., et al. (2003). "Depression and coronary heart disease in women with diabetes." *Psychosomatic Medicine,* vol. 65, pp. 376–383.

Goodnick, P., et al. (1997). "Sertraline in coexisting major depression and diabetes mellitus." *Psychopharmacology Bulletin,* vol. 33, pp. 261–264.

Lustman, P., et al. (1998). "Cognitive behavior therapy for depression in type 2 diabetes mellitus: A randomized, controlled trial." *Annals of Internal Medicine,* vol. 129, pp. 613–621.

Lustman, P., et al. (2001). "Association of depression and diabetes compli-cations." *Psychosomatic Medicine,* vol. 63, no. 4, pp. 619–630.

Lustman, P., et al. (2001). "The prevalence of comorbid depression in adults with diabetes." *Diabetes Care,* vol. 24, no. 6, pp. 1069–1078.

Van Tilberg, M. A. L., et al. (2001). "Depressed mood is a factor in glycemic control in type 1 diabetes." *Psychosomatic Medicine,* vol. 63, pp. 551–555.

HOSTILITY

Lane, J. D., et al. (2000). "Personality correlates of glycemic control in type 2 diabetes." *Diabetes Care,* vol. 23, pp. 1321–1324.

Niaura, R., et al. (2002). "Hostility and the metabolic syndrome in older males: The Normative Aging Study." *Psychosomatic Medicine,* vol. 62, pp. 7–16.

Räikkönen, K., et al. (2003). "Hostility predicts metabolic syndrome risk factors in children and adolescents." *Health Psychology,* vol. 22, pp. 279–286.

Stabler, B., et al. (1987). "Type A behavior pattern and blood glucose control in diabetic children." *Psychosomatic Medicine,* vol. 49, pp. 313–316.

Surwit, R. S., et al. (2002) "Hostility, race, and glucose metabolism in non-diabetic individuals." *Diabetes Care,* vol. 25, pp. 835–839.

WEIGHT LOSS

Allen, H. N., and Craighead, L. (1998). "A cognitive behavioral intervention for binge eating." *Cognitive and Behavioral Practice,* vol. 2, no. 2, pp. 249–270.

Allen, H. N., and Craighead, L. W. (1999). "Appetite monitoring in the treatment of binge eating disorder." *Behavior Therapy,* vol. 30, pp. 253–272.

RELAXATION TECHNIQUES

Lane, J. D., et al. (1993). "Relaxation training for non-insulin dependent diabetes: Predicting who will benefit." *Diabetes Care,* vol. 16, pp. 1087–1094.

Surwit, R. S., et al. (1978). "A comparison of cardiovascular biofeedback, neuromuscular biofeedback, and meditation in the treatment of borderline essential hypertension." *Journal of Consulting and Clinical Psychology,* vol. 46, no. 2, pp. 252–263.

Surwit, R. S., et al. (1983). "The effects of relaxation on glucose tolerance in non-insulin-dependent diabetes." *Diabetes Care,* vol. 6, no. 2, pp. 176–179.

Surwit, R. S., et al. (1984). "Relaxation-induced tolerance is associated with decreased plasma cortisol." *Diabetes Care,* vol. 7, no. 2, pp. 203–204.

Surwit, R. S., et al. (2002) "Stress management improves long-term glycemic control in type 2 diabetes." *Diabetes Care,* vol. 25, no. 1, pp. 30–34.

Takuya, T., et al. (2002) "The effect of qi-gong relaxation exercise on the control of Type 2 diabetes mellitus." *Diabetes Care,* vol. 25, pp. 241–242.

DRUG INTERACTIONS

Lane, J. D., et al. (1993). "Relaxation training for non-insulin dependent diabetes: Predicting who will benefit." *Diabetes Care,* vol. 16, pp. 1087–1094.

Lane, J. D., et al. (2003). "Caffeine impairs glucose tolerance in type 2 diabetes." *Diabetes,* vol. 54, Suppl. 1 (abstract).

Lustman, P., et al. (1995). "Effects of alprazolam on glucose regulation in diabetes: Results of a double-blind, placebo-controlled trial." *Diabetes Care,* vol. 18, pp. 1087–1094.

Surwit, R. S., et al. (1986). "Alprazolam reduces stress hyperglycemic in ob/ob mice." *Psychosomatic Medicine,* vol. 48, pp. 278–282.

Surwit, R. S., et al. (1989). "Differential glycemic effects of morphine in diabetic and normal mice." *Metabolism,* vol. 38, pp. 282–285.

Thong, F., et al. (2002). "Caffeine-induced impairment of glucose tolerance is abolished by beta-adrenergic receptor blockage in humans." *Journal of Applied Physiology,* vol. 92, pp. 2347–2352.

Van Dam, R., et al. (2002). "Coffee consumption and risk of type 2 diabetes mellitus." *Lancet,* vol. 360, pp. 1477–1478.

Acknowledgments

No scientific or medical contribution ever comes from only one individual. Any contributions I have made are largely due to my work with others. I acknowledge the help of many people who contributed to helping me understand the mind-body connection with diabetes through personal interaction and collaboration or through their independent work, which served as both an inspiration and source of knowledge. In particular, I recognize the following individuals:

- Mark Feinglos, M.D., who introduced me to the problem of stress and diabetes and has collaborated with me on almost all of the work I have done in this field
- Richard Johnson, Ph.D., who first introduced me to the link between physiology and psychology and is responsible for my pursuing a career in psychology
- Ernest Poser, Ph.D., who taught me how to be both a clinician and a researcher
- Donald Hebb, Ph.D., a pioneer and giant in the field of brain-behavior research, who taught me what it means to be a scientist
- David Shapiro, Ph.D., who introduced me to the area of mind-body medicine and served as my most important mentor in the development of my scientific career
- Herbert Benson, M.D., whose pioneering work on the relax-

ation response brought the idea that stress management could be used as a medical treatment

- Redford Williams, M.D., who served as both a mentor and colleague in my early years at Duke University and who encouraged me to follow my instincts in pursuing the mind-body connection in diabetes
- Linda Craighead, Ph.D., who provided assistance in developing the section on appetite awareness training
- Nancy Zucker, Ph.D., for her help with the section on cognitive behavior therapy
- Leslie Meredith, Dorothy Robinson, Edith Lewis, and others at Free Press for their belief in this project, their careful eyes, and their constructivee feedback. Your insight and advice helped transform the raw manuscript into a much better book.

I also acknowledge the support I have received from the National Institutes of Health, the American Diabetes Association, and the John D. and Katherine T. MacArthur Foundation. These organizations provided funding for most of the research on which this book is based.

Finally, I acknowledge and thank my wife, Sandra, and my children, Daniel and Sarah, for the love and support that I depend on and without which this book would not have been possible.

Index

Homeostasis, 29
Hostility, 51–61, 120
    caffeine and, 220, 222, 223
    causes of, 59–60
    cognitive behavior therapy for,
        65, 72, 97, 99, 101–2, 108–9
    depression and, 55, 59, 60
    diabetes link to, 56–58
    disease risk and, 58–59
    help for, 60–61
    serotonin and, 30, 55, 59–60
    support systems and, 58, 117–18
    testing level of, 71–72
Hostility syndrome, 58, 60
    antidepressants and, 227–28, 229
    components of, 54–55
Hunter, John, 55
Hyperinsulinemia, 8, 10, 15, 17
Hypertension, 3, 9. *See also* Blood
        pressure
    hostility and, 57, 58
    metabolic syndrome and, 7
    progressive muscle relaxation
        and, 75
    relaxation techniques and, 25, 74
    stress and, 52
Hypothalamus, 20, 26, 28, 29, 55, 83

If-then beliefs, 112
"Ignore fullness" cycle, 207–8
"Ignore hunger/too hungry" cycle, 207
Imipramine (Tofranil), 47, 228
Immune system
    depression and, 49
    mind control of, 23
    type 1 diabetes and, 6, 7, 30, 40
Impotence, 9
Incontinence, 9
India, 11
Insulin, 6, 75. *See also* Hyperinsu-
        linemia; Insulin resistance
    alcohol and, 226
    antianxiety medication and, 231
    antidepressants and, 229
    caffeine and, 221
    depression and, 46
    discovery of, 11, 29
    epinephrine and, 27
    exercise and, 19
    fat burners and, 232
    green tea and, 222

    hostility and, 57, 58, 59
    obesity and, 201
    stress and, 26, 30, 36, 40
    type 1 diabetes and, 7
    type 2 diabetes and, 7–8
Insulin resistance, 6–7, 230
    basic information on, 8
    caffeine and, 221
    defined, 6
    depression and, 41, 46
    fat and, 17
    hostility and, 57, 58
    stress and, 27
    thrifty genotype and, 13, 15
Irritable bowel syndrome, 28
Islets of Langerhans, 6

Jacobson, Edmund, 80
James, Henry, 37
Johns Hopkins University, 44
Jordan, Michael (quoted), 143
*Journal of the American Medical
        Association,* 48

Kabat-Zinn, Jon, 241
Kaiser Permanente Center for Health
        Research, 44
Kidney disease, 8, 9, 17

Labeling, 111
Lactate levels, 235
Lancet, 221
Lane, James, 220, 221
Latin Americans, 14
Lennon, John (quoted), 124
Leonardo da Vinci (quoted), 122
Leptin, 13
Life expectancy, 10
Lifestyle factors, 12–13, 16–17, 204
Lincoln, Abe (quoted), 125
Livingston, Elizabeth, 35–36
Low-fat diets, 17–18, 60–61
Lustman, Patrick, 47, 49, 99, 228

MacLaine, Shirley (quoted), 130
Maharishi Mahesh Yogi, 235
Maharishi University of Management,
        235, 249

Valium, 231
Venlafaxine (Effexor), 229
Vipassana, 241
Virgin Islands, 58

Washington University School of
        Medicine, 47, 49, 99, 228
Weight gain. *See also* Obesity;
        Overeating
    alcohol and, 225
    antidepressants and, 47, 228, 229
    antihistamines and, 232
Weight loss, 17–19. *See also* Appetite
        awareness
    antidepressants and, 229
    programs for, 250–51
    realistic goals for, 204
Wellbutrin (bupropion), 229–30
West, Mae (quoted), 151
Western Electric, 56
"What the heck" cycle, 208
Wilde, Oscar (quoted), 155
Williams, Redford, 54, 60, 61

Willis, Thomas, 20
Winfrey, Oprah (quoted), 191
Withdrawal
    from antianxiety medication, 231
    from caffeine, 223
    from nicotine, 224, 225
Women
    depression in, 29, 48
    heart disease risk in, 9, 48
    thrifty genotype in, 13
Wright, Frank Lloyd (quoted), 169
Written observations. *See also* Food
        diary; Six-week planner
    in cognitive behavior therapy,
        105, 106, 107, 114
    in disclosure therapy, 243–45

Xanax, 231

Zoloft (sertraline), 229
Zyban (bupropion), 224, 225, 229–30

ABOUT THE AUTHORS

RICHARD S. SURWIT, PH.D., is Professor and Vice Chairman of the Department of Psychiatry and Behavioral Sciences and Chief of the Division of Medical Psychology at Duke University Medical Center in Durham, North Carolina. The author of more than one hundred studies on diabetes, metabolism, and stress, he is the cofounder of the Duke Neurobehavioral Diabetes Program and jointly runs the Behavioral Endocrinology Clinic at Duke, which has extensively studied the role that emotions and personality play in blood sugar control.

Dr. Surwit is recognized as a world authority on diabetes and stress. He is past president of the Society for Behavioral Medicine and is the recipient of a Research Scientist Career Award from the National Institute of Mental Health. His research has been funded by the National Institutes of Health for more than twenty years. His work has been praised by experts across the country, including current and past presidents of the American Diabetes Association.

Dr. Surwit's scholarly writing has been published in leading scientific journals, including *Nature, Diabetes, Diabetes Care, American Journal of Physiology, Journal of Clinical Investigation, Metabolism, Psychosomatic Medicine,* and *Endocrinology,* as well as in popular magazines, including *Psychology Today* and *Men's Health.* He has appeared on national television shows such as *Good Morning America, CBS Evening News, Fox News,* and *CNN's Mid-Day Report.* He speaks regularly at large annual conferences such as the American Diabetes Association, the American Psychological Association, and the Society for Behavioral Medicine.

ALISA BAUMAN is a professional writer whose work has appeared in *Better Homes & Gardens, Prevention, Runner's World, Men's Health, Builder,* and *Walking* magazines. She is a certified yoga instructor and regular columnist for *Yoga Journal* magazine. Her previous books include *Fat to Firm at Any Age* and *Fight Fat: Secrets to Successful Weight Loss.*